Clinical Handbook of Yamamoto New Scalp Acupuncture

of related interest

Vibrational Acupuncture
Integrating Tuning Forks with Needles
Mary Elizabeth Wakefield and Michel Angelo
Foreword by Donna Carey
ISBN 978 1 84819 343 7
eISBN 978 0 85701 299 9

The Principles and Practical Application of Acupuncture Point Combinations
David Hartmann
Foreword by John McDonald
ISBN 978 1 84819 395 6
eISBN 978 0 85701 352 1

Acupuncture for Headaches, Eyes and ENT Pathologies
Hamid Montakab
ISBN 978 0 85701 404 7
eISBN 978 0 85701 405 4

Neuropuncture
A Clinical Handbook of Neuroscience Acupuncture, Second Edition
Michael D. Corradino
Foreword by Giovanni Maciocia
ISBN 978 1 84819 331 4
eISBN 978 0 85701 287 6

Clinical Handbook of Yamamoto New Scalp ACUPUNCTURE

David Bomzon
with
Avi Amir

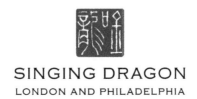

SINGING DRAGON

LONDON AND PHILADELPHIA

First published in 2020
by Singing Dragon
an imprint of Jessica Kingsley Publishers
73 Collier Street
London N1 9BE, UK

www.singingdragon.com

Library of Congress Cataloging in Publication Data
A CIP catalog record for this book is available from the Library of Congress

British Library Cataloguing in Publication Data
A CIP catalogue record for this book is available from the British Library

ISBN 978 1 84819 392 5
eISBN 978 0 85701 350 7

Printed and bound in Great Britain

Contents

* * * * * *

Acknowledgments

• • • • • •

Many people have contributed to the writing of this book over the years: our teachers of traditional Chinese medicine, our families, the staff in our clinic, our students, our colleagues, and our patients. Although these contributions were sometimes made without the individuals knowing that they had contributed, we thank them all for their support, their questions, and their insights. We have learnt a great deal from them during our 12 years of practice and the last two years while writing this book.

We would like to acknowledge the contribution of Lionel (Arieh) Bomzon, David Bomzon's father. Two years ago, when we were approached to write this book and were very hesitant and thinking to say "no thank you," he was the one who pushed us to accept the offer and the challenge. We are also aware that it was very exasperating and maddening as an editor, who is not familiar with the theory and practice of traditional Chinese medicine and acupuncture, to transform our words and ideas into lucid, concise, and easy-to-understand English for the reader's benefit. Thank you!

This book could have not come into being without recognizing the contribution of Dr Toshikatsu Yamamoto, the discoverer and developer of this amazing and wonderful method of acupuncture, namely Yamamoto New Scalp Acupuncture (YNSA). He was our teacher of YNSA and repeatedly reminded us that the most important thing in being a practitioner is the patient: "the more the practitioner knows this method then the more the patients will benefit from it." Thank you—we have been privileged to be your students.

Last, but not least, we acknowledge the loving support of our wives, Racheli Bomzon and Inna Amir. You were, and still are, the wind in our sails because this book could not have been written without your support.

Thank you for being there and for giving us a shoulder to rest on. We have never taken you for granted and feel privileged to be married to you. We love you with all our hearts.

●　　●　　●　　●　　●

This book is dedicated to my children, Itmar, Yotam and Eliya, and all children with learning difficulties. If you put your mind to it and you really want something, your dreams can come true. Believe in yourself.

Preface

● ● ● ● ● ●

This book was initially a handout to participants in our workshops that we delivered in Israel and other countries. Over time, we added more information to it until it came to a stage that we were ready to publish it as a clinical handbook on Yamamoto New Scalp Acupuncture (YNSA). In this book, we will be presenting our understanding and expertise on YNSA. In doing so, we thank Dr Toshikatsu Yamamoto, the discoverer and developer of YNSA, for first teaching and then guiding us on YNSA in his seminars and courses in which we participated in Miyazaki, Japan.

When I began my career several years ago as an inexperienced and young Chinese medicine practitioner, I was always seeking new ways to improve the treatments for my patients and provide rapid relief of their symptoms. In my search for knowledge and more tools to treat neurological patients, I stumbled across YNSA, which, in those days, was a very new and unfamiliar method of acupuncture in Israel. After seeing a stroke patient with right-sided paralysis move after my colleague, Gil Kotler, needled some of the basic points of YNSA, I decided to learn more about it. At first, Gil began to teach me about YNSA and I then became his teaching assistant in the workshops that he was giving in Israel. After some time, I decided to travel to Japan in order to attend one of Dr Yamamoto's seminars on YNSA. After my return from Japan, Gil retired and I began teaching YNSA to practitioners in Israel with the belief that more practitioners would begin to use YNSA, and that their patients would therapeutically benefit from this treatment. In addition to applying YNSA to patients in my clinic, I began applying it to patients in the rehabilitation department of Bnei Zion Medical Center, Haifa, Israel. In this department I initiated a collaborative research program to investigate the effects of YNSA on the rehabilitation of stroke patients and other patients with neurological disorders.

As a Chinese medicine practitioner, I continued to look for an explanation of YNSA's mode of action in Chinese medicine terminology in order to improve my understanding of it. At the time, the theoretical basis of YNSA was based on western medicine's understanding and practice of neurology. In my search, I was hoping that I could bring a new understanding to the method and enable more Chinese medicine practitioners to understand YNSA, thereby making the method comprehensible. I therefore began my partnership with Avi Amir, one of my former YNSA students, who is a massage therapist and acupuncturist. As co-author of this book, Avi brings a slightly different approach on the application of YNSA. After incorporating Avi's knowledge, the reader will have a broader view on YNSA.

Before writing this book, we read many other books written on YNSA and found that there is not much information on the location of the needling points. We have therefore catalogued the location of all the needling points so that the reader can easily locate them when applying YNSA. We also wanted to accurately describe all the groups of needling points and provide an understanding of how to use a specific group.

We present our experiences as a result of managing a successful clinic and treating more than 150 patients a week with YNSA and acupuncture since 2009. Participants of our teaching workshops on YNSA asked many questions, such as: What is the location of the needling points? What are the indications for needling a specific point? We have included case studies from our clinic in order to improve the practitioner's understanding of YNSA, and in adding such examples we hope to reinforce the foundations of YNSA.

Introduction to Modern Scalp Acupuncture

• • • • • •

Chinese scalp acupuncture is primarily considered to be a modern acupuncture method and can be described as an amalgam of western medical knowledge of the cerebral cortex and traditional Chinese needling techniques. In addition to its proven effectiveness in the treatment of chronic disorders of the central nervous system, Chinese scalp acupuncture is known for its immediate delivery of positive results, despite using fewer needles than in body acupuncture.

One of the scalp acupuncture methods developed in the late 20th century was Yamamoto New Scalp Acupuncture (YNSA). Before describing YNSA in detail, I will first present a brief history of scalp acupunc-ture because this was the essence for developing YNSA.

History of scalp acupuncture

Acupuncture is a traditional method of treatment in oriental medicine. It has been in use for more than 2500 years and has evolved into a unique and effective treatment. Due to modern knowledge and technology being integrated into traditional oriental medicine, new acupuncture techniques have continued to emerge, notably laser and electrical acupuncture, as well as the discovery of new acupuncture points. Judging by its evolution, continuous development, and effectiveness, it is safe to label scalp acupuncture as the most significant breakthrough that can be credited to Chinese acupuncture since the 1970s.

Although the new discoveries and developments in acupuncture can be attributed to extensive clinical experience, the use of acupuncture for treating neurological disorders can be traced back to the early years of Chinese civilization. For instance, the earliest and most important written work on Chinese acupuncture, *Huang Di Nei Jing* (*The Yellow Emperor's Classic of Internal Medicine*), was published in 100 BCE: this text describes in detail the links between the brain and the body with regard to physiology, pathology, and treatment, according to available evidence during this period.

In the 1950s, contemporary Chinese scalp acupuncture began to receive significant attention in terms of research and development. Specifically, renowned Chinese physicians and neurologists began in-depth investigations into the relationship between the human brain and the body, and integrated the existing knowledge of neurophysiology into traditional Chinese medicine. For example, Professor Fan Yunpeng sketched a prone homunculus on the scalp, with the head directed towards the forehead and the legs directed towards the occipital region (see Figure 0.1). Professor Tang Song-yan sketched two homunculi on the scalp, with the first in a supine position and the second in a recumbent position (see Figure 0.2). The scalp acupuncture methods of Professors Yu Zhi-shun and Zhang Ming-qing comprise acupuncture points that are located on the channels or meridians on the head. Professor Zhu Ming-qing also formulated new and multiple special therapeutic zones on the scalp (see Figures 0.3 and 0.4).

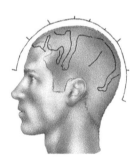

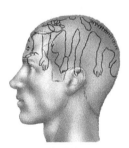
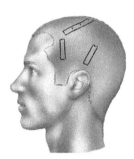

FIGURE 0.1   FIGURE 0.2   FIGURE 0.3

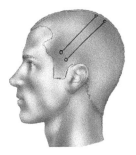
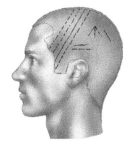
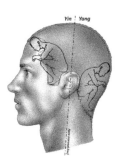

FIGURE 0.4   FIGURE 0.5   FIGURE 0.6

It took about two decades for Chinese acupuncturists to integrate their knowledge on brain functions into the principles of traditional Chinese medicine.

Dr Jiao Shun-fa is widely regarded as the founder of Chinese scalp acupuncture. He combined traditional Chinese acupuncture methods with modern-day knowledge of neurophysiology and neuroanatomy to develop a major new tool that influences the function of the central nervous system (see Figure 0.5).

Following a detailed investigation and testing of Dr Shun-fa's discovery, scalp acupuncture was later formally recognized and acknowledged by the acupuncture profession when it was included in the 1977 edition of *Acupuncture and Moxibustion*, a national acupuncture textbook. Scalp acupuncture was recognized internationally in 1987 when it was described at the First International Acupuncture and Moxibustion Conference in Beijing, China. Although the use of scalp acupuncture at that time was limited to the treatment of aphasia caused by stroke and paralysis, its use has expanded and evolved extensively due to advanced research and extensive clinical experience.

The treatment of different central nervous system disorders using scalp acupuncture has yielded positive results, especially in cases of pain and paralysis that stem from chronic neurological disorders.

In 1973, a Japanese anesthesiologist, Dr Toshikatsu Yamamoto, discovered a new microsystem on the scalp that he named YNSA; his theory was based on a combination of western knowledge of neurology and traditional oriental medicine (see Figure 0.6).

Unlike scalp acupuncture, which is comprised of needling zones, YNSA comprises 60 needling points, which are divided into five groups.

In YNSA, the points are usually needled ipsilateral to the side of the symptoms and diagnostic zones, scalp acupuncture, where the needling zones are needled contralateral to the side of the symptoms.

While in scalp acupuncture, manipulation of the needle is necessary once the needle is inserted into the needling zone, Dr Yamamoto believed that it is not necessary in YNSA because any movement by patients causes the needle to be manipulated.

Nowadays, YNSA is considered to be the most modern and most developed method of scalp acupuncture that exists.

General principles of scalp acupuncture

Since scalp acupuncture is based on western medicine and neurological knowledge, most of the needling zones are located on the scalp and are equivalent to their anatomical location in the brain. Their function is based on the corresponding or equivalent of the brain. For example, for a patient suffering from paralysis of the hand, the zone that will be needled is the zone on the scalp that is equivalent to the location of the motor hand area of the hand on the brain.

Here are some further examples: The indication for needling the Du-20 acupuncture point is to treat paralysis of the foot. Since the Du-20 acupuncture point is located on the scalp, we will see that it is equivalent to the location of the foot's anatomical area in the brain.

One of the indications for needling the GB-19 acupuncture point is to treat vertigo and loss of balance. This point is located on the occipital bone and is equivalent to the anatomical location of the cerebellum.

The indication for needling the Yin Tang extra acupuncture point is insomnia, and this point matches the anatomical location of the pituitary gland in the brain.

The Chinese medical practitioners who developed the scalp acupuncture method were able to think outside the box: they understood that the brain is constantly changing and is able to make new synaptic connections. This ability is called neuroplasticity in western medical science. This concept was 50 years ahead of its time because it was believed that the brain develops and changes only during childhood and that any loss of brain function after childhood due to injury could not be restored. Only 25 years ago brain scientists started to understand that the brain continues to make new synaptic connections, even after childhood. Many traditional Chinese medical practitioners believed that neurological disorders could be treated by scalp acupuncture by stimulating the damaged regions of the brain.

In scalp acupuncture, the zone to needle is determined according to the patient's symptoms, and the main diagnosis carried out according to the practitioner's knowledge of western medicine. Once the practitioner has chosen the zone to needle, the needle is inserted contralaterally at a 15–30° angle into the subcutaneous tissue of the scalp and threaded through the connected tissue fibers in the specific needling zone. Once the needle is in place, the practitioner can manipulate the needle manually or using an electrostimulation device. For example, the foot zone on the left side of the scalp can be needled to treat a patient with paralysis of the right foot due to a stroke in the left hemisphere of the brain. This zone will be needled because it corresponds to the anatomical location of the foot in the brain.

1

Introduction to Yamamoto New Scalp Acupuncture (YNSA)

• • • • • •

Dr Toshikatsu Yamamoto, a Japanese physician and scientist, found an independent acupuncture system in the 1960s. At the Japanese Ryodoraku Congress in Japan in 1973, Dr Yamamoto reported his acupuncture system, which initially comprised five acupuncture points, for the first time. He named these points the "basic points," and found needling them was very effective in treating people who had had strokes, were experiencing pain, or were paralyzed. In addition to auricular acupuncture and Sujok acupuncture (a Korean hand acupuncture microsystem), YNSA has become the most widely practiced form of microsystem acupuncture at the present time. Since the original report in 1973, many other needling points, such as the dorsal somatotopes (points located on the spine), brain points, sensory points, Ypsilon (organ) points, and cranial points, and several diagnostic zones in the neck, abdomen, and elbow, have been discovered.

Dr Yamamoto continues to search and discover new acupuncture points and somatotopes on the scalp in his daily work, in his quest to use scalp acupuncture for treating pain.

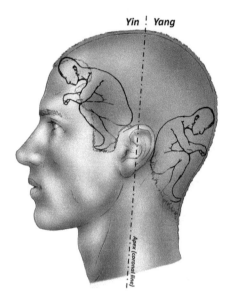

FIGURE 1.1

Principles of YNSA

Nowadays, the five basic points are the most commonly used needling points in YNSA. In the early years of YNSA, these points were needled ipsilaterally to the side on which the patient was experiencing pain. In contrast, the brain points, which were developed later, were needled contralaterally to the side on which the patient was experiencing pain.

With ongoing development of YNSA, the five basic points subsequently expanded into nine basic points, and a specific diagnostic zone for each basic point was discovered in the neck and elbow regions (discussed later in the book). Currently, the selection of basic points to needle and the needling side are done according to the sensitivity of the neck, abdomen, and elbow diagnostic zones (discussed later in the book).

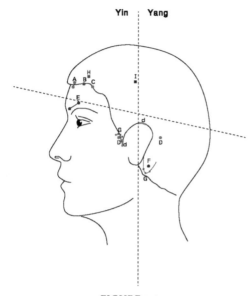

FIGURE 1.2

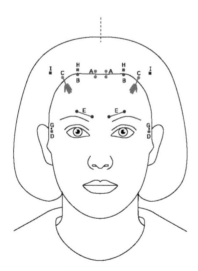

FIGURE 1.3

YNSA is considered to be a conventional form of acupuncture and the entire body is depicted on the scalp. It is one of many types of micro-system acupuncture, such as the auricular, nasal, and hand microsystems (microsystems acupuncture is based on the belief that small and specific areas on the body correspond to all organs and parts of the body). The internal organs are depicted by 12 Ypsilon (internal organ) points, which are located on the temporal muscle, and the 12 cranial nerve points, which are located on the anterior part of the epicranial aponeurosis.

The 12 Ypsilon points have two somatotopic locations: one on the anterior temporal muscle (Yin aspect of the scalp) and the other on the posterior part of the temporal muscle (Yang aspect of the scalp).

YNSA has unique diagnostic zones in the neck, which are related to the 12 Ypsilon points and the 12 cranial nerve points. When there is a disorder of a channel or an organ, the specific diagnostic point in the neck will be sensitive when palpated.

A pressure-sensitive point (diagnostic point) is located on the neck or abdomen, while a related treatment point (needling point) is located on the temporal muscle. These 12 needling points (12 Ypsilon needling points) also represent the 12 traditional Chinese medicine channels (meridian) and organs. When the practitioner finds sensitivity in a diagnostic point, it means that a channel, meridian, or organ is not functioning well. By needling the corresponding point that is associated with that specific diagnostic zone, the practitioner is treating the organ and channel that is not functioning well.

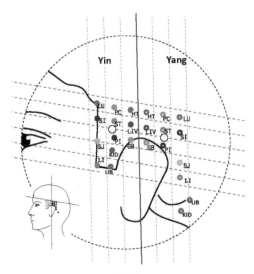

FIGURE 1.4

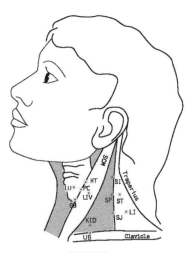

FIGURE 1.5

When, for example, the practitioner finds that the Kidney diagnostic zone in the neck diagnostic zone is sensitive, the practitioner will then needle the KID Ypsilon point or KID cranial nerve point. Once the KID Ypsilon or cranial nerve point is accurately needled, the sensitivity of the Kidney diagnostic zone in the neck will wane, and this provides instant affirmation that the correct point was needled (discussed later in the book).

YNSA's needling points are divided into several categories, all of which are located on the Yin and Yang aspects of the scalp.

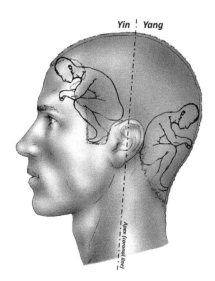

FIGURE 1.6

The five groups of needling points of YNSA

- Nine basic points, which are named A, B, C, D, E, F, G, H, and I. Needling or stimulation of these points exerts an extensive effect on the internal organs, musculoskeletal system, and peripheral nervous system. Five of the basic points, namely the A, B, C, D, and E points, are located on the forehead on either side of the midline along the natural hairline on the Yin aspect. The basic E point is located above both eyebrows in the supraorbital foramen. The F point is unusual because it is located in the occipital area behind the ears over the mastoid process of the temporal bone at the height of the ear's tragus on the Yang aspect. The H and I points were added after discovery of the A, B, C, D, E, F, and G points, and the I point has since become a somatotope. Eight of the nine points, namely the A, B, C, D, E, F, G, and H points, have reflection symmetry in the occipital area on the Yang aspect of the scalp.

- Four facial sensory points, which are named the eye, nose, mouth, and ear points (see Figure 1.7). These are located on both sides of the face and also have reflection symmetry on the Yang aspect of the scalp. Three of these sensory points, namely the eye, nose, and mouth points, are located bilaterally on the forehead in an area between the basic A and E points (about 1 cm lateral to the midline, below the location of basic point A and the medial area of point E). The ear point is located at the continuation of point C towards the bridge of the nose and at a height that is between and lateral to the eye and nose points. Needling one of these points medicates the sense and muscles of that facial sensory organ.

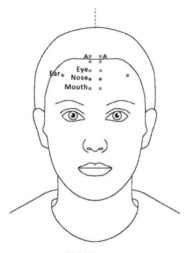

FIGURE 1.7

- Three brain zones (points), which are named the cerebrum, cerebellum, and basal ganglia (midbrain) points (see Figure 1.8). These are located bilaterally close to the scalp's mid sagittal line just above the frontal hairline on the Yin and Yang aspects of the scalp. Needling or stimulation of these points exerts an effect on the central nervous system.

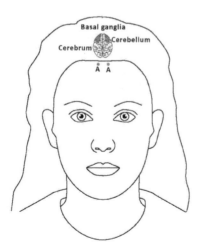

FIGURE 1.8

- Twelve Ypsilon points, which are named KID, UB, LU, SI, PI (Spleen/Pancreas), ST, SJ, LI, GB, PC, HT, and LIV (see Figure 1.9). These points are bilaterally located in the temporal region of the scalp on the Yin and Yang aspects. Needling or stimulation of these points exerts an effect on the 12 internal organs and 12 meridians.

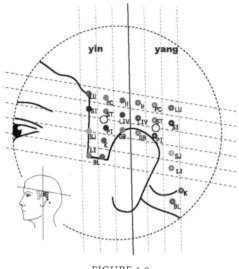

FIGURE 1.9

- The twelve cranial nerve points, which are located bilaterally and are a posterior continuation of the basic A point, are a linear constellation of eight tiny points (see Figure 1.10). Six of these 12 points overlie the brain points. Needling or stimulation of these points exerts effects on the internal organs.

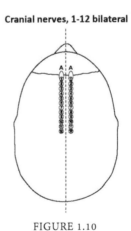

FIGURE 1.10

Most of these points are associated with a diagnostic zone, which should be palpated before selecting the needling point and the body side to be needled because an accurate diagnosis improves the therapeutic value of the acupuncture treatment.

The choice between needling on the Yin and Yang aspects

All the points that are located on the Yin (anterior) aspect of the scalp are also located on the Yang (posterior) aspect of the scalp.

Approximately 95 percent of treatments rely on needling points on the Yin aspect of the scalp. The exceptions are those needling points that are on the Yang aspect of the scalp, such as the G point, which is needled for chronic problems of the knee, and the F point, which is needled for sciatic pain. The F point on the Yin aspect is not needled because it is not functional.

The easiest way of selecting the correct Yang point to needle is to first palpate the corresponding points on the Yang and Yin aspects of the scalp, and then needle the most sensitive of the two points.

For example, a patient complains of neck pain and the practitioner finds that the basic A point on the left side must be needled. After palpating the cervical diagnostic zone in the elbow, the practitioner will then palpate and compare the sensitivity of the basic A point on the Yin and Yang aspects of the scalp, and the most sensitive point of the two will be needled. Other examples include:

- When the Kidney diagnostic zone on the neck is very sensitive and the scalenus anterior muscle is soft or flaccid when palpating the area (the muscle is not resistant to palpation) (see Figure 1.11). *Note: When the Kidney diagnostic test zone is sensitive and the muscle is resistant to palpation, this would be an indication to needle points on the Yin aspect.*

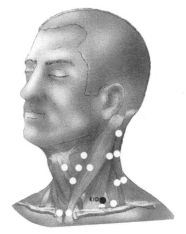

FIGURE 1.11

- When treatment on the Yin aspect does not relieve symptoms and/or there is no response.

- When treating patients with multiple sclerosis (MS).

- When treating neurodegenerative diseases in which demyelination occurs.

- When treating all tremors, irrespective of their cause, such as Parkinson's disease and essential tremor. For treating rigidity in patients with Parkinson's disease, the needling points on the Yin aspect are preferred. There are also circumstances when points on the Yin and Yang aspects are needled concomitantly.

How YNSA works

Although it is recommended that an acupuncture needle should be inserted at a 15° angle, the direction and angle of insertion is not important. It is very important, however, that the needle's tip reaches the sensitive point on the scalp.

The needling points on the scalp are located in the loose connective tissue below the subcutaneous tissue of the scalp's skin. They are bumps or granules whose size is not more than 1 mm, feel like mustard seeds, and are sensitive when palpated (see Figure 1.12).

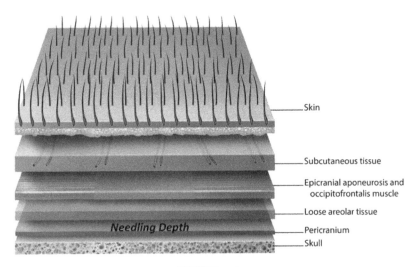

FIGURE 1.12

Needle stimulation during or after acupuncture is not necessary.

For acute disorders, the duration of needling is from 1 minute to 20 minutes. For chronic disorders, the duration of needling is from 30 minutes to up to one hour. In some cases, it is recommended that the patient is sent home after insertion of the intradermic needles, depending on the effect the practitioner wants to achieve and the severity of the patient's condition.

The acupuncture needles that Dr Yamamoto recommends and uses are violet-colored Seirin 0.25 mm (diameter) x 40 mm (length). Although we usually use 20 mm x 30 mm needles, we found that any type of acupuncture needle is effective as long as the needle's tip reaches a sensitive area.

The number of weekly treatments can differ from patient to patient, and it depends on how much stimulation the practitioner wishes to give. In chronic cases, it can range from two to three treatments a week for about five weeks. In acute cases, it can range from one to two treatments a week over three weeks.

Laser acupuncture is very effective when treating elderly patients and young children. When used, it is recommended to apply the laser beam at a 30° angle. Dr Yamamoto has also used a helium–neon laser as an alternative to needling in children and very nervous patients with an acute condition.

Electrostimulation can also be considered for improving clinical outcomes. Dr Yamamoto proposed that electrostimulation could possibly be used for treating very long-standing chronic conditions.

Acupressure and massage can be applied to the needling point instead of acupuncture, and is recommended for use in infants and young children. When acupressure and massage is used, each point should be massaged for at least 2–3 minutes.

Diagnostic zones

The diagnostic zones for needling points on the Yin and Yang aspects are the same, and most points are needled according to the sensitivity of their diagnostic zones. The diagnostic zones for the basic A, D, E, F, I, and brain points are located very close to the Kidney diagnostic zone in the neck, as well as in the cubital fossa or the inside of the elbow (crook of the elbow). The diagnostic zones of the 12 Ypsilon and 12 cranial nerve points are located in the neck and abdomen.

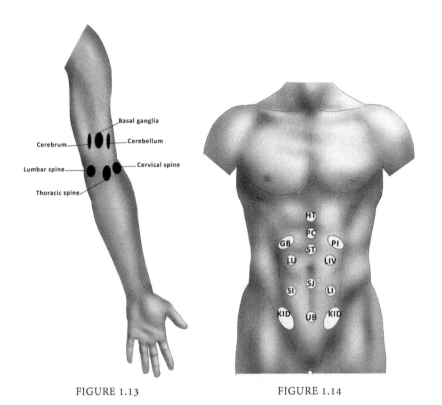

FIGURE 1.13   FIGURE 1.14

How to use the diagnostic zones

Most treatments comprise an initial palpation of the diagnostic zones followed by needling of a specific point. There are three diagnostic zones: the neck, abdominal, and elbow. The sensitivity of a diagnostic zone will determine which point will be needled. The sensitivity and tension of the muscle in the neck and abdominal diagnostic zones will determine which Ypsilon and cranial nerve points should be needled. The sensitivity of the elbow diagnostic zone will determine which spinal and brain points will be needled. After inserting the needle, the diagnostic zone is palpated again in order to check whether the sensitivity of the diagnostic zone has been lessened.

Note: According to traditional Chinese medicine, a channel or meridian is a concept (simplified Chinese: 经络; traditional Chinese: 經絡; pinyin: jīngluò, also called channel network) through which the life-energy known as "qi" (in western terms this can be translated as "function") flows. Each organ is associated with a longitudinal anatomical pathway that runs through different parts of the body. Each channel or meridian possesses a specific physiological function.

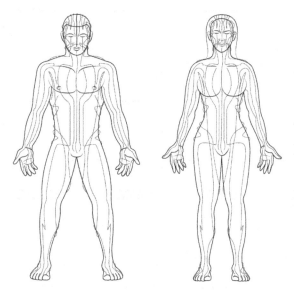

FIGURE 1.15

How to palpate the diagnostic zones

Palpation of a diagnostic zone is done using the upper third of the thumb, slowly applying increasing pressure that should not exceed 1 kg (2.2 lbs). Take a scale so that you can appreciate what 1 kg (2.2 lbs) pressure is. When palpating a specific diagnostic zone, apply pressure slowly around the zone and increase the pressure so that it does not exceed 1 kg (2.2 lbs) when examining for sensitivity and tension in the zone. In order to obtain the most objective input from the zone, the goal is to detect sensitivity or tension by applying the least pressure possible.

The patient can respond to palpation in four ways:

- The patient says, "I feel the pressure but no sensitivity." In this case, the practitioner will not needle the corresponding needling point that is associated with the specific zone. For example, when the patient says this while the practitioner is palpating the cervical diagnostic zone in the elbow, the practitioner will not needle the corresponding point in the scalp.

- The patient says, "I feel slight pressure and slight sensitivity." In this case, the practitioner may choose to needle the corresponding point.

- The patient says, "I feel pain and sensitivity." In this case, the practitioner may choose to needle the corresponding point.

- The patient says, "It is very painful and sensitive," and instinctively withdraws the hand when the practitioner is palpating the diagnostic zone. In this case, the practitioner may choose to needle the corresponding point.

Note: When needling, the practitioner should always start with those points that are associated with the most sensitive diagnostic zone. The practitioner should also check the other zones that are less sensitive than the most sensitive zone. Before needling a specific point that is associated with the less sensitive zones, the practitioner should also palpate the less sensitive zones. Only if they are still sensitive will the practitioner needle the specific needling point that is associated with the less sensitive zones.

For example, the practitioner finds that the cervical diagnostic zone in the patient's elbow on the right arm is very sensitive, and the lumbar diagnostic zone on the left arm is only slightly sensitive. Accordingly, the practitioner first needles the basic A point on the right side. Before needling the basic D point on the left side, the lumbar diagnostic zone in the elbow on the left arm is palpated for the second time. If the practitioner finds that the lumbar diagnostic zone in the elbow is no longer sensitive, there is no need to needle the basic D point.

2

The Basic Points

· · · · · ·

The basic points comprise nine points, namely A, B, C, D, E, F, G, H, and I, and are named so because they were the first points that Dr Yamamoto discovered and were the basis for YNSA's subsequent development and expansion. YNSA was established by repeated trial and error, and the C point was the first point Dr Yamamoto discovered. After its discovery, he discovered another six points, namely the A, B, D, E, F, and G points. A few years later, he discovered another two points, H and I, which he incorporated into the basic points. In recent years, the I point has become a vital point for treating pain. This point has developed into a complete somatotope that covers the entire body.

The basic points are constructed in a manner that each point covers and treats a different region of the body and the nearby organs that are located in that region. The basic points slice the body into a series of horizontal and vertical planes that cover the body from the skin inwards and from the head down to the feet. If a disorder is caused by an emotional imbalance, the preferred needling points are the Ypsilon points (discussed later). The basic points are needled to alleviate all types of musculoskeletal pain, which exerts an effect on the body's kinetic system and modifies the balance of the surrounding organs. Initially, Dr Yamamoto needled these basic points and obtained very good results when treating pain and various kinetic disorders in specific regions of the body. For example, needling the A point will resolve a neck and head problem, but will also affect the larynx, vocal cords, and thyroid gland.

Using pain as an example, remember that it can be experienced physically and emotionally or psychologically. Needling the basic points will help treat physical pain. If the pain is not lessened after treatment, it is possible that the emotional component will need to be treated. For this purpose, the practitioner might choose to needle the Ypsilon points.

General overview of the basic points

- A: The area between the head and cervical spine from C1 to C7.

- B: The area between the neck and shoulder.

- C: The area between the shoulder and the palm of the hand.

- D: The area of the lumbar spine from the diaphragm to the feet.

- E: The area of the thoracic spine from T1 to T12.

- F: The area of the buttocks (gluteal muscles).

- G: The area of the knee.

- H: Extra-lumbar point 2, the lower extremities, and the knee.

- I: Extra-lumbar point 3, a complete somatotope that covers the entire body.

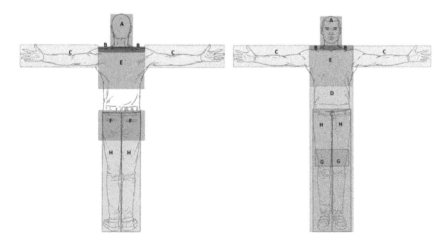

FIGURE 2.1

All basic Yin points are located on the frontal hairline of the skull, and the basic Yang points are a mirror reflection of the Yin points around the occipital sutures on the Yang aspect. The location of each point can change according to the anatomy of the patient's scalp and skull. In Chinese medicine, the word "jun," which means "relative scale," is used to describe the location of points. In YNSA, the word "approximately" is used because the location of each point in each region is imprecise and can change because of the patient's anatomy. The needling points in YNSA on patients with a wide and high forehead are located more distally or laterally. For patients with a narrow skull and a small forehead, the needling points will be close to each other and have a small diameter.

The correct location of a point can be identified as an indentation or a minute protrusion (a small granule like a mustard seed beneath the skin), which is sensitive and/or painful when pressure is applied to the point. The location of the points can also change when the patient has scars on the scalp. These scars can reposition the points slightly lateral or medial to the point's usual location. This repositioning not only occurs with the basic points, but also with all points in the system.

Although the points are sensitive, the practitioner needs to feel granules beneath the skin. The practitioner's knowledge of the location of a specific point will still require the practitioner to confirm the exact location of each point by testing for sensitivity and feeling the granules.

With experience, Dr Yamamoto was able to locate each point using his fingertips to palpate the scalp. In order to confirm a point's location, Dr Yamamoto applied pressure at different locations in order to make the patient aware of the different sensations when pressure was applied at the correctly located point.

When needling a basic point, the needle is subcutaneously inserted until the patient experiences the sensation of a small electric shock. After insertion, the needle's final position may have to be adjusted a little in order to locate the exact spot and achieve the best therapeutic result. If the expected therapeutic outcome is not realized and YNSA is discontinued, any subsequent poor results are attributed to failure in properly locating the correct therapeutic points.

Diagnostic areas of the basic points

Some basic points have a diagnostic area that is located in the elbow region. The sensitivity of the diagnostic area will dictate the choice of which point to needle. The diagnostic zones in the elbow are palpated bilaterally. Needles are inserted into the specific needling point ipsilateral to the sensitive side in the elbow diagnostic zone.

For example, a 34-year-old man presents with cervical pain. The diagnostic area in the elbow that is associated with the cervical spine (area of the lateral epicondyle) on both sides (left elbow and right elbow) should be palpated. The A point should be needled on the same side according to the sensitivity of the diagnostic area in the elbow region (see Figure 4.3).

Using the basic points for obtaining maximum therapeutic benefit

Proficiency in the use of the basic points requires an understanding of the entire kinetic chain and the musculoskeletal system, the nervous system, and the functions of the internal organs. The clinical results will be good when a practitioner is familiar with the kinetic chain and the musculoskeletal system.

The selection of the needling points on each side is done according to the sensitivity in the diagnostic zone (elbow, neck, or abdomen).

For example, the diagnostic zone of the cervical spine is located in the left and right radial elbow region. The sensitivity of the diagnostic zone will determine which point and side will be needled. This selection process for a needling point and side will be repeated for the thoracic region and lumbar region. After needling the point, the practitioner should check whether the sensitivity in the elbow region has subsided. If the sensitivity has diminished, it means that the correct point was needled.

The first stage of treatment is diagnosis in either the elbow or the neck region and then needling the appropriate basic points. This approach enables treatment of the problem's source. When palpating the needling zones (the basic needling zones are A, C, and E, and the basic needling points are B, D, extra D, F, G, and H), the practitioner will needle the most sensitive point in the zone.

For example, the A point is a 2 cm line on which several sensitive points are located. Therefore, the most sensitive point will be needled first.

When palpating a zone or point, the practitioner needs to think of it as "digging for treasure"—the coordinates are known, and the practitioner should look for the precise location of the sensitive granules. Sometimes the practitioner might have to go a few millimeters to the left or a few millimeters to the right, or in the superior or inferior directions, to locate the point before needling it.

The basic points can be also used for symptomatic treatment. For example, a patient complains of an ongoing migraine. Point A on the same side as the migraine or bilaterally can be needled to relieve it (the A point can be needled on both sides without taking into account the side of the head where the migraine is sensed). If a patient complains of lower back pain on the right side, the D point can be needled according to the symptoms without making a diagnosis. In this case the D point is needled on the side of the lower back pain.

When needling a point, some patients will often feel a strong stinging sensation, which can last for approximately 10 seconds before it subsides and can be likened to being hit on the head with a small hammer.

Case examples for needling the basic points

Example 1: A patient complains of pain in the left shoulder. According to the sensitivity of the diagnostic zone of the lumbar region on the right side, something is possibly tugging the quadratus lumborum muscle on the right side, which may be causing the shoulder pain. Needling the basic D point (needling the basic D point will treat the lumbar spine) will treat the region of the neck and shoulder, and by doing so the shoulder pain will subside. In this case, the cause of the pain was the spasm in the quadratus lumborum muscle that manifested as increased sensitivity in the lumbar diagnostic zone in the elbow. In this case, the D point was needled ipsilateral to the side of the elbow diagnostic zone of the lumbar spine that was sensitive.

Example 2: A 35-year-old five-week pregnant woman complains of nausea, vomiting, and heartburn. The symptoms of the heartburn originate from the area of the thoracic spine that corresponds to the area of the basic

E point. In this case, needling the E point bilaterally will be therapeutically beneficial, even though there is no indication for needling this point in order to treat the heartburn and the other symptoms. After needling this point, the patient is relieved of all the symptoms.

Example 3: An 18-year-old man complains of itching around the neck on the right side. The A point on the right side was needled because this point covers the neck region. After needling the A point, the itching was relieved within 12 hours.

Dr Yamamoto also reported that asthma and angina, two conditions of the internal organs, could be successfully treated by needling the basic E point bilaterally and always by needling the lung Ypsilon point.

It is highly recommended that the practitioner becomes experienced in needling the basic points before needling the Ypsilon and cranial nerve points. Needling the Ypsilon and cranial nerve points requires knowledge of the abdominal and neck diagnostic zones, and the indications for their needling are more complex than those required for needling the basic points. *Note: The diagnostic zones in the neck and abdomen require a more experienced hand when locating and palpating the sensitivity in the diagnostic zone, because they are more difficult to locate.*

In general, a practitioner should try to use a minimum number of needles—even needling one basic point can bring relief to a patient. The more knowledge a practitioner has on the musculoskeletal anatomy, the better the practitioner can focus the treatment and use the minimum number of needles.

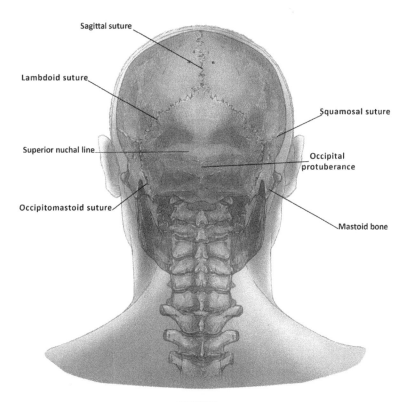

FIGURE 2.2

Locations and indications for needling the basic points

Although the indications for needling each basic point are listed in the table at the end of Chapter 4, I found that the indications for needling each point are more extensive than those described by Dr Yamamoto. Additionally, there are two considerations that will allow the practitioner to keep an open mind when selecting the optimal points to needle so that the therapeutic outcome will be maximal. The first is the area in the body that each point depicts, and the second is the indication for needling a particular point. Of the two considerations, the area is more important than the specific indications for needling of the point.

Basic point A

Yin location: The point is located on a 2 cm vertical line that runs from 1 cm above the hairline (A1=C1 spine) to 1 cm below the hairline (A8=C8 spine). This 2 cm line is located approximately 1 cm lateral to the sagittal line (see Figures 2.3, 2.4, and 2.5).

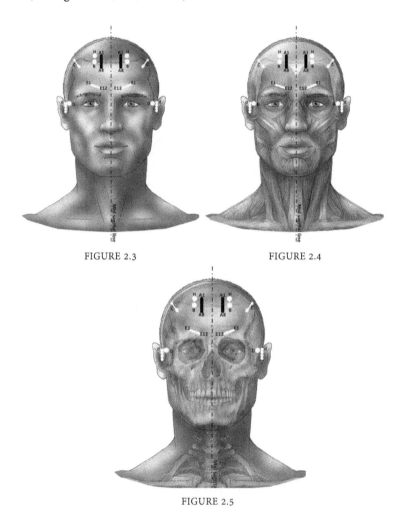

FIGURE 2.3   FIGURE 2.4

FIGURE 2.5

Yang location: The point is located on a 1.5 cm vertical line that runs from 0.75 cm above the lambdoid suture to 0.75 cm below the lambdoid suture. This line is located approximately 0.75 cm lateral to the mid-sagittal line (0.75 cm lateral to the Du-19 acupuncture point or the point where the lambdoid and sagittal sutures meet) (see Figure 2.6).

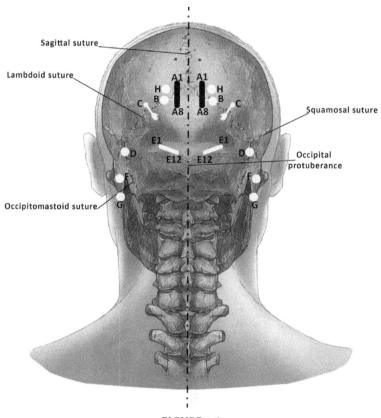

FIGURE 2.6

Yin and Yang indications:

- Any type of neck pain
- Whiplash
- Laryngitis
- Skin lesions on the neck
- Headaches or any type of migraine
- Vertigo
- Facial paralysis
- Neck paralysis
- Trigeminal neuralgia
- Thyroid disorders
- Aphasia
- Voice loss
- Disorders of the sensory organs (eye, nose, mouth, and ear)
- Toothache

Basic point B

Yin location: The point is located on the anterior natural hairline approximately 2 cm lateral to the mid-sagittal line of the face/head (see Figures 2.7, 2.8, and 2.9).

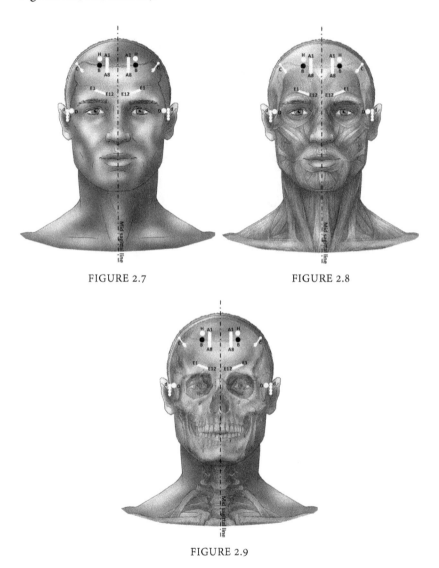

FIGURE 2.7   FIGURE 2.8

FIGURE 2.9

Yang location: The point is located on the lambdoid suture and approximately 1.5 cm lateral to the mid-sagittal line (see Figure 2.10).

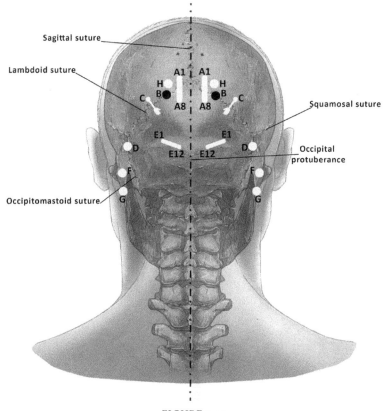

FIGURE 2.10

Yin and Yang indications:

- Thyroid and parathyroid disorders

- Any disorder in the area between the supraclavicular fossa and the supraspinatus fossa

- Scalene myofascial pain syndrome

- Shoulder pain and arm paralysis

- Frozen shoulder

- Hemiplegia of the shoulder

- Lower neck pain

- Spasm of the trapezius muscle, which will cause headaches

Basic point C

Yin location: The point is located on a line that begins 1 cm above the hairline and continues 1 cm below the hairline at an approximate angle of 45° to the nasal bridge. The mid-point of this 2 cm line is the GB-13 acupuncture point (on the superior border of the temporalis muscle) (see Figures 2.11, 2.12, and 2.13).

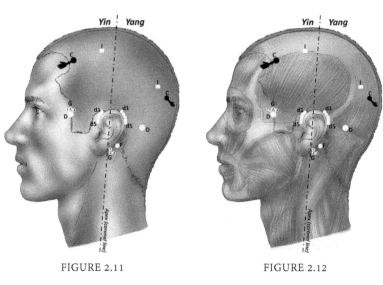

FIGURE 2.11   FIGURE 2.12

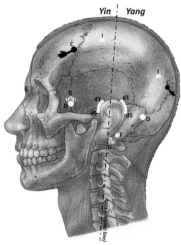

FIGURE 2.13

Yang location: The point is located on a 1.5 cm oblique line that runs from 0.75 cm above the lambdoid suture to 0.75 cm below the lambdoid suture.

This line is located approximately 3.5 cm lateral to the mid-sagittal line. To locate this needling point, take a 45° angle from the external occipital protuberance towards the lambdoid suture, and the point is located where this line meets the lambdoid suture (see Figure 2.14).

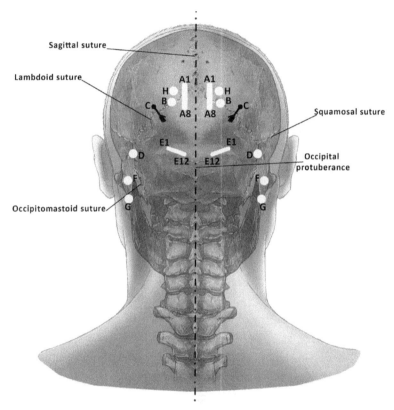

FIGURE 2.14

Yin and Yang indications:

- Paralysis of the hand and the whole arm
- Arm and hand ataxia
- Tremor of the hand or arm
- Carpal tunnel syndrome
- De Quervain's tenosynovitis
- Trigger finger

- Golf elbow/tennis elbow
- Rheumatic arthritis of all the joints of the shoulder/elbow, palm of the hand, and wrist joints
- Bursitis
- Multiple sclerosis
- Parkinson's disease

Basic point D

Yin location: The point is located on the front hairline (sideburn) on a line which connects the root of the ear and the outer canthus of the eye (see Figures 2.15, 2.16, and 2.17).

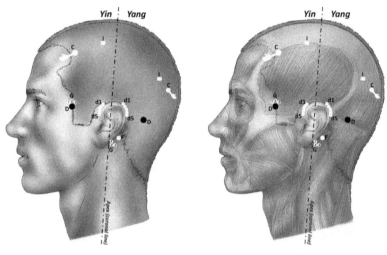

FIGURE 2.15   FIGURE 2.16

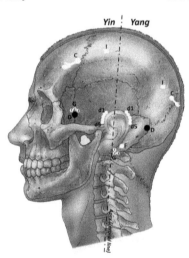

FIGURE 2.17

Yang location: The point is located on the occipitomastoid suture at the same level as the lower border of the upper third of the ear (see Figure 2.18).

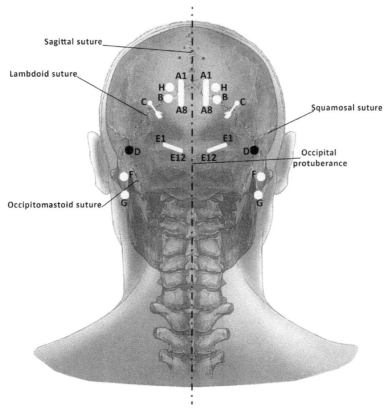

FIGURE 2.18

Yin and Yang indications:

- Lower back pain with radiation to the lower extremities
- Paralysis of the lower extremities and the lower abdomen
- Premenstrual syndrome
- Lower abdomen pain
- Diarrhea and constipation
- Urinary tract infections
- Gynecological disorders
- Nausea and vomiting
- Parkinson's disease which affects the lower extremities
- Multiple sclerosis (MS) which affects the lower extremities
- Ankle sprains and fractures
- Gout
- Spasticity of the lower extremities
- Prolapsed disc

- Herniated disc
- Rheumatic arthritis of any joint from the lower back down to the feet (hip, knee, ankle, and toes)

Basic point extra D

Yin location: The point is located just below the ear base where the face meets the ear (see Figures 2.19, 2.20, and 2.21).

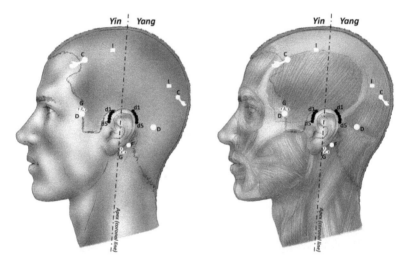

FIGURE 2.19   FIGURE 2.20

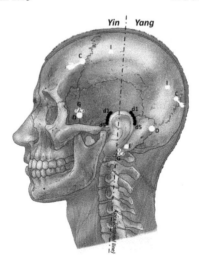

FIGURE 2.21

Yang location: The point is located on the uppermost edge of the mastoid bone (see Figure 2.22).

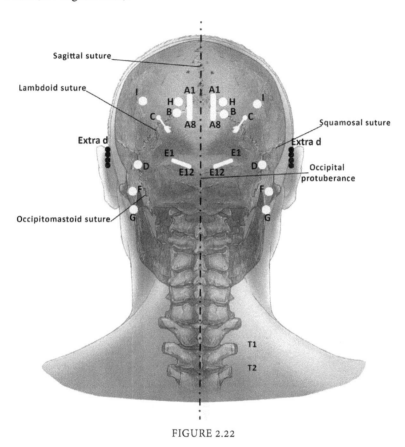

FIGURE 2.22

Yin and Yang indications:

- Lower back pain
- Sciatica
- Anal pain
- Lumbago

Basic point E

Yin location: The point is located on an oblique 2 cm line that starts 1 cm lateral to the midline above the eyebrow (see Figures 2.23, 2.24, and 2.25).

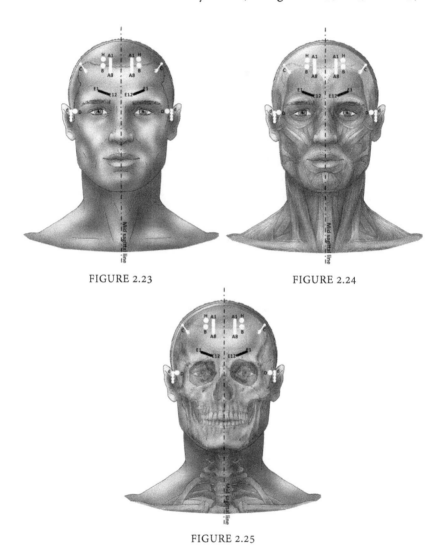

FIGURE 2.23   FIGURE 2.24

FIGURE 2.25

Yang location: The point is located on a crest above the superior nuchal line on a 2 cm horizontal line that runs from 3 cm lateral to the mid-sagittal line to approximately 1 cm lateral to the mid-sagittal line (see Figure 2.26).

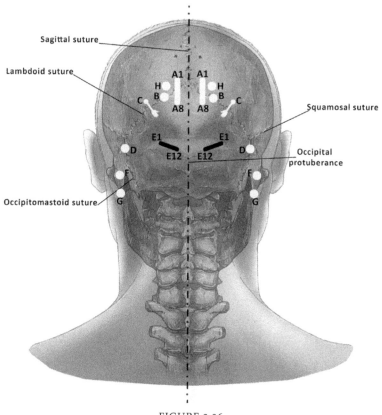

FIGURE 2.26

Yin and Yang indications:

- Intercostal neuralgia
- Herpes zoster
- Fractures
- Angina pectoris
- Palpitations
- Asthma
- Dyspnea
- Bronchitis

- Bradycardia and tachycardia
- Bradypnea and apnea
- Heartburn
- Dyspepsia
- Gastroesophageal reflux disease
- Nausea and vomiting

Basic point F

Yin location: The F point does not have a location on the Yin aspect.

Yang location: The point is located on the highest point of the mastoid bone.

Note: The point is at the same level as the lower tragus of the external ear.

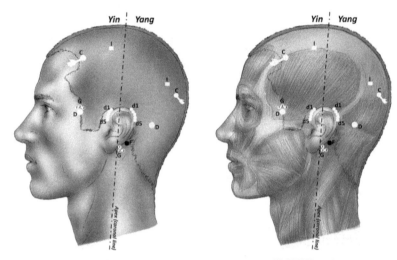

FIGURE 2.27   FIGURE 2.28

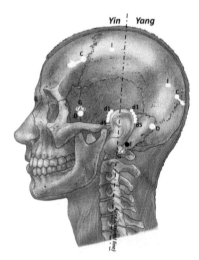

FIGURE 2.29

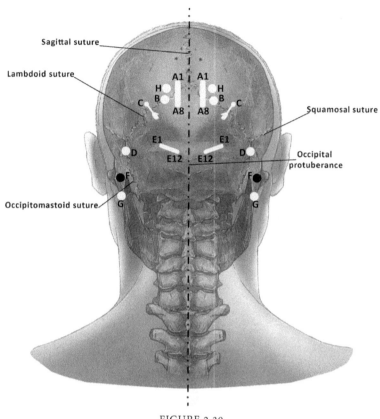

FIGURE 2.30

Yin and Yang indications:

- Lower back pain
- Any disorder in the area of the gluteus maximus
- Piriformis syndrome
- Sciatica
- Hemorrhoids and anal fissures

Basic point G

Yin location: The point is located in the arch about 3 mm above the D point (see Figures 2.31, 2.32, and 2.33).

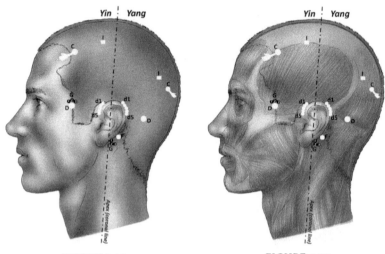

FIGURE 2.31   FIGURE 2.32

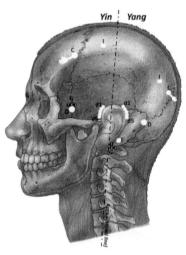

FIGURE 2.33

Yang location: The point is located on the edge of the mastoid bone (SJ-17 acupuncture point) (see Figure 2.34).

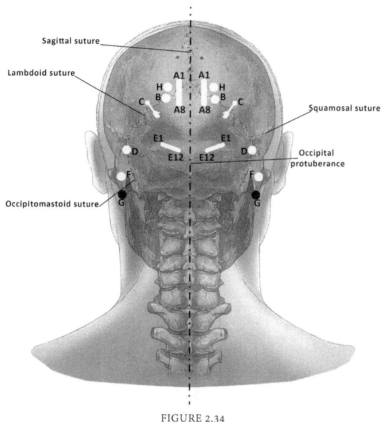

Sagittal suture

Lambdoid suture

Squamosal suture

Occipital protuberance

Occipitomastoid suture

FIGURE 2.34

Yin and Yang indications:

- Rheumatic arthritis of the knee
- Arthritis of the knee
- Bursitis of the knee
- Patella fractures and patella arthritis
- Baker's cyst (located at the back of the knee)
- Meniscus disorders of the knee

Note: The G Yin basic point is needled for treating acute knee pain, and the G Yang basic point is needled for treating chronic knee pain.

Basic point H

Yin location: The point is located approximately 1 cm above the basic B point (see Figures 2.35, 2.36, and 2.37).

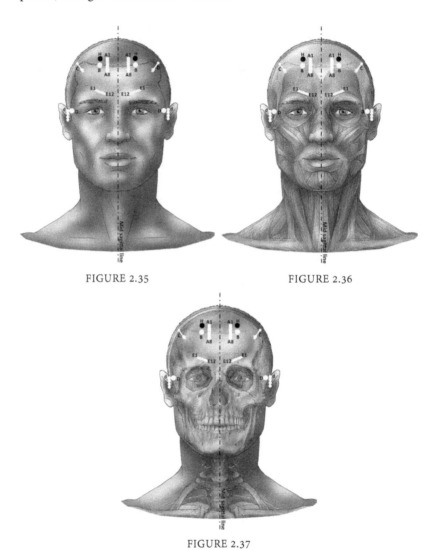

FIGURE 2.35   FIGURE 2.36

FIGURE 2.37

Yang location: The point is located approximately 0.75 cm above the basic B Yang point (see Figure 2.38).

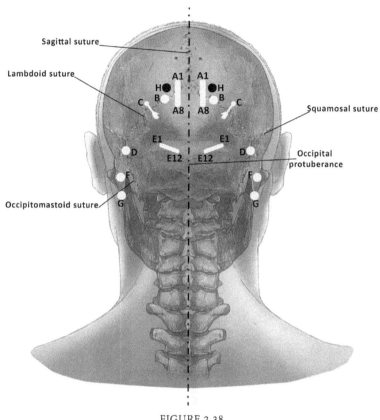

FIGURE 2.38

Yin and Yang indications:

- Any disorder of the lower extremities from the hip down to the ankle (it is more effective for treating balance and equilibrium)

- Bow-legged or knock-kneed posture

- Knee pain due to bad alignment and posture of the legs

- Lower back pain that radiates down to the feet

- Imbalance and instability

Basic point I

Yin location: The point is located approximately 2–3 cm anterior to the apex line and approximately 4 cm above the apex of the ear.

Yang location: The point is located approximately 2–3 cm posterior to the apex line and approximately 4 cm above the apex of the ear.

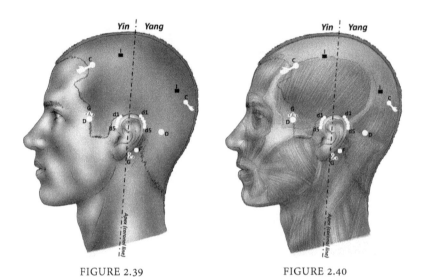

FIGURE 2.39   FIGURE 2.40

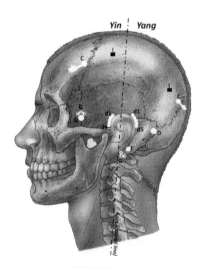

FIGURE 2.41

Yin and Yang indications:

- To augment the effect of needling the D point

- Sciatica

- Lumbago

- Weakness of the lower extremities

- Paralysis of the lower extremities

In recent years, the I point, which is located in the temple region just above the ear, has become a very significant point of treating pain and has developed into a whole somatotope in its own right. Nowadays, the I somatotope covers the whole body, and needling this point exerts an effect on the entire body (see Figure 2.42).

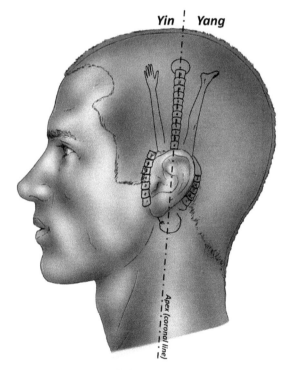

FIGURE 2.42

3

Brain Zones and Sensory Organ Points

• • • • • •

Brain zones

There are three brain zones, namely the cerebral, cerebellum, and basal ganglia zones.

The diagnostic zones of the brain are located in the elbow region and in the abdomen. Needling the brain zones exerts an effect on the central nervous system. For example, needling the cerebral zone can affect mood, hormonal secretions, and the sensory and motor cortices, and needling the cerebellum zone can affect motor coordination and fine motor skills. The function of the basal ganglia zone is to control voluntary motor movements.

Locations and indications for needling the brain zones
Cerebral zone

Yin aspect: This zone is located approximately on a 2 cm vertical line that runs from 1 cm to 3 cm into the hairline. This line is located approximately 1 cm lateral to the mid-sagittal line (sagittal suture) (see Figure 3.1).

Note: The superior part of the basic A point line overlaps the inferior part of the cerebral zone. Other books on YNSA state that the cerebral zone is located 1 cm superior to the basic A point.

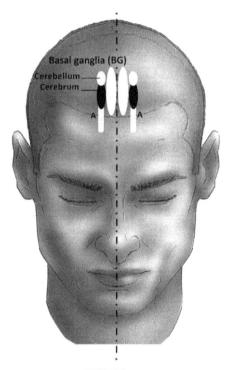

FIGURE 3.1

Yang aspect: This zone is located approximately on a 1.5 cm vertical line that runs from approximately 0.75 cm above the lambdoid suture up to approximately 1.5 cm above the lambdoid suture. This line is located approximately 0.75 cm lateral to the mid-sagittal line (sagittal suture) (see Figure 3.2).

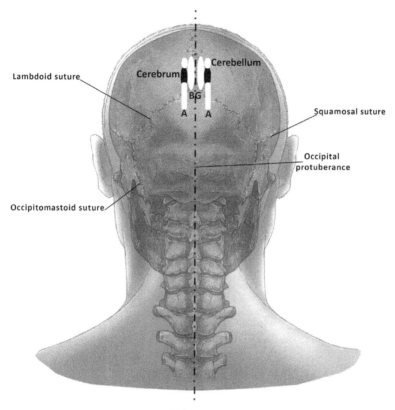

FIGURE 3.2

Yin and Yang indications:

- Chronic pain
- Acute pain
- Neuropathic disturbances
- Motor and sensory disturbances
- Hemiplegia and paraplegia
- Migraines and headaches (cluster and tension headaches)
- Trigeminal neuritis
- Dementia
- Insomnia
- Multiple sclerosis (MS)
- Depression and psychological disturbances
- Hormonal disturbances
- High and low blood pressure
- Memory loss
- Attention deficit disorder (ADD)
- Attention deficit hyperactivity disorder (ADHD)
- Aphasia
- Visual disturbances

Cerebellum zone

Yin aspect: This zone is located approximately on a 1 cm vertical line that runs from 3 cm to 4 cm into the hairline. This line is located approximately 1 cm lateral to the mid-sagittal line (sagittal suture) (see Figure 3.3).

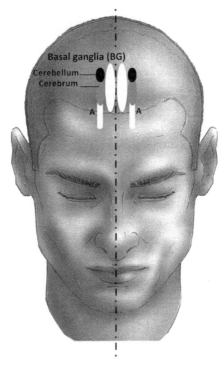

FIGURE 3.3

Yang aspect: This zone is located approximately on a 0.75 cm vertical line that runs from 1.5 cm to 2.25 cm above the lambdoid suture. This line is located approximately 0.75 cm lateral to the mid-sagittal line (sagittal suture) (see Figure 3.4).

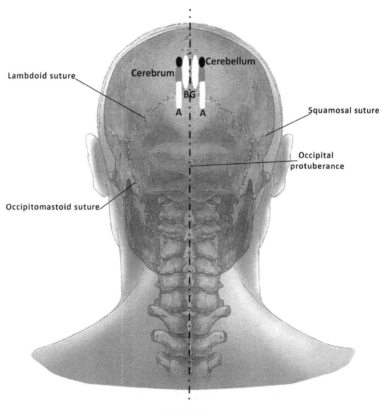

FIGURE 3.4

Yin and Yang indications:

- Balance disturbances
- Vertigo and dizziness
- Ataxia
- Proprioceptive disturbances
- Learning disorders
- Chronic pain
- Nociception
- Visual and auditory processing
- Dystonia
- Tremors
- Gastrointestinal disturbances

Basal ganglia zone

This zone has two locations: an old location, based on the abdominal diagnostic zone around the xiphoid process of the sternum, and a new location, based on the elbow diagnostic zone.

Yin aspect of the old location: The old location of the zone is located approximately on a 3 cm vertical line that runs from 1 cm to 4 cm into the hairline. This line is located on the mid-sagittal line (sagittal suture) (see Figure 3.5). The old location is used when the practitioner cannot use the elbow for the diagnosis.

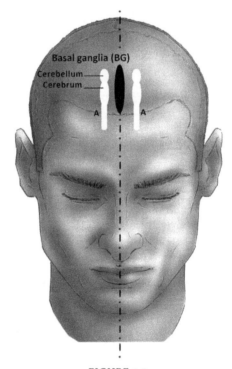

FIGURE 3.5

Note: This line can start on the hairline and can extend to approximately 5 cm into the hairline. Other books state that the location is on a line that begins approximately 1 cm into the hairline up to approximately 5 cm into the hairline.

Yang aspect of the old location: The old location of the zone is located approximately on a 3 cm vertical line that runs from 1 cm to 4 cm above the lambdoid suture. This line is located on the mid-sagittal line (sagittal suture) (see Figure 3.6).

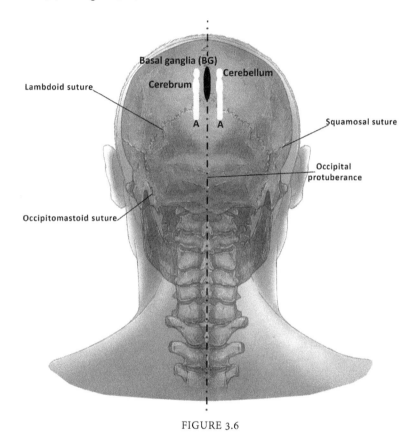

FIGURE 3.6

Yin aspect of the new location: The new location of the zone is located approximately on a 3 cm vertical line that runs from 1 cm to 4 cm into the hairline. This zone is located approximately 0.5 cm lateral to the mid-sagittal line, midway between the A line and the mid-sagittal line (see Figure 3.7).

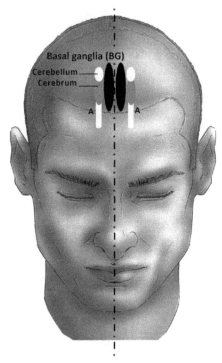

FIGURE 3.7

Yang aspect of the new location: The new location of the zone is located approximately on a 2.5 cm line that runs from 0.75 cm to 3.25 cm above the lambdoid suture. This line is located between the A line on the Yang aspect and the sagittal suture (see Figure 3.8).

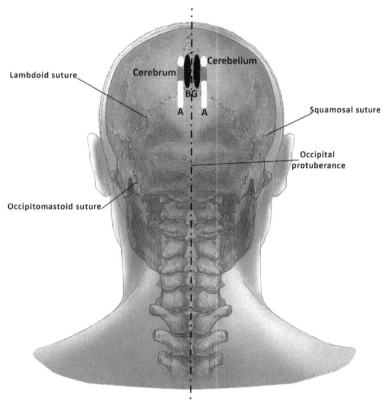

FIGURE 3.8

Yin and Yang indications:

- Rigidity
- Tremors
- Involuntary movement disorders
- Restless legs syndrome
- Parkinson's syndrome and Parkinson's disease

- Chronic pain
- Depression
- Movement disorders (hyperkinetic disorders)
- Huntington's disease
- Dystonia
- Hemiballismus

Sensory organ points

The sensory organ points comprise four points that are located on the face and were discovered after discovery of the basic points. These are named according to the organ that each point represents, namely the eyes, nose, mouth, and ears. The manner in which each point is detected and needled is the same as that described for the basic points. Specifically, the practitioner should first search for the sensitive area before needling the point. For example, if a patient complains of a mouth problem, the practitioner should first search for the sensitive area in the mouth and then needle the mouth sensory point.

The four sensory points are located on the forehead, and in the Yang region on the occipital bone. The eye, nose, and mouth sensory points are located at an equal distance between the inferior border of the basic A zone and the middle border of the basic E zone on the Yin and Yang aspects of the scalp. Additionally, the Yang sensory points are mirror-reflected on the occipital bone.

The sensory points have no diagnostic zones, and needling of these points is done on the same side as the affected organ. For example, the ear point on the right-hand side is needled for treating pain in the right ear. For inflammation of the eye on the right-hand side, the eye point on the right-hand side is needled.

Needling a particular sensory point affects the sensory and motor (all the muscles around the sense) functions of that sense. For example, facial palsy is a condition where the mouth or eye muscles are paralyzed and the affected patient may not be able to close or shut one eye. Although needling the eye point can help the patient shut the affected eye, needling this point will affect vision and the sensory-motor function of the eye muscles. Additionally, needling the eye point will be useful for treating paralysis of the eyelid, pain around the eye, and irritability of the eye, as well as visual disorders due to a cataract, diplopia, or glaucoma.

The practitioner should also note that needling the basic A point will also influence the four sensory points.

Locations and indications for needling the sensory organ points

Eye point

Yin aspect: The point is located approximately 1 cm below the inferior part of the basic A point (see Figures 3.9, 3.10, and 3.11).

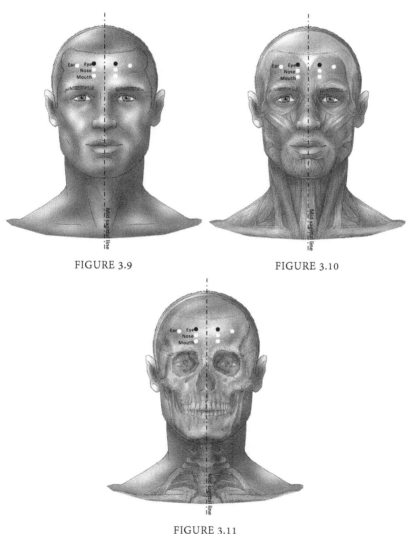

FIGURE 3.9

FIGURE 3.10

FIGURE 3.11

Yang aspect: The point is located on the occipital bone approximately 1 cm below the inferior part of the basic A point (see Figure 3.12).

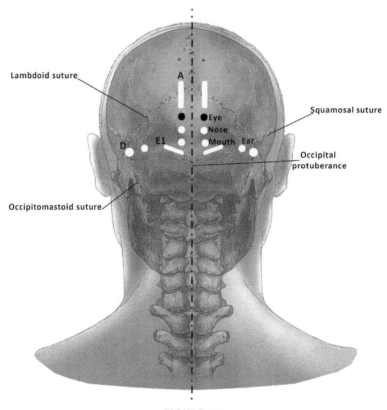

FIGURE 3.12

Yin and Yang indications:

- All ophthalmic disturbances and pain
- Inflammation
- Itching
- Redness
- Loss of vision

- Glaucoma
- Cataract
- Lazy eye
- Dryness of the eye
- Loss of function of the muscles that surround the eye

Nose point

Yin aspect: The point is located approximately 2 cm below the line of the A point in the middle of the forehead (see Figures 3.13, 3.14, and 3.15).

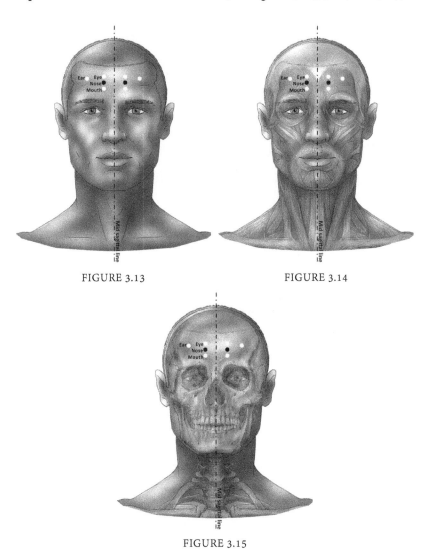

FIGURE 3.13   FIGURE 3.14

FIGURE 3.15

Yang aspect: The point is located on the occipital bone approximately 2 cm above the midpoint of the line of the E point (see Figure 3.16).

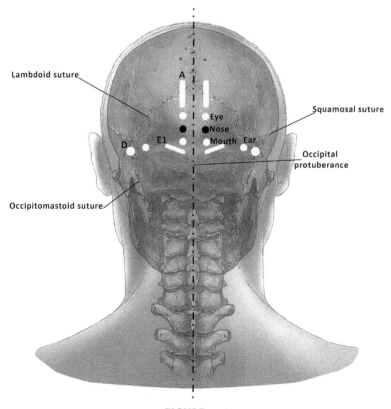

FIGURE 3.16

Yin and Yang indications:

- Loss of smell
- Nasal polyps
- Sinusitis
- Rhinitis

- Nasal congestion
- Running nose
- Allergies

Mouth point

Yin aspect: The point is located approximately 1 cm above the midpoint of the line of the E point (see Figures 3.17, 3.18, and 3.19).

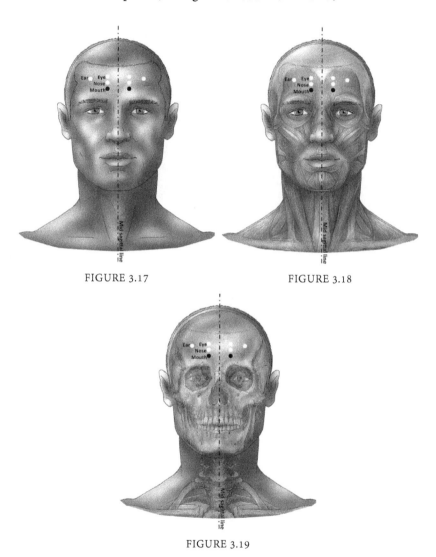

FIGURE 3.17

FIGURE 3.18

FIGURE 3.19

Yang aspect: The point is located on the occipital bone approximately 1 cm above the midpoint of the line of the E point (see Figure 3.20).

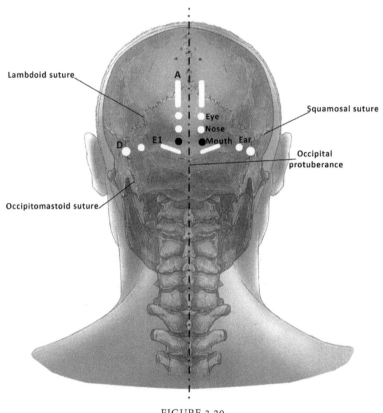

FIGURE 3.20

Yin and Yang indications:

- Speech problems

- Motor aphasia

- Toothache

- Inflammation and infections of the oral cavity

- Oral ulcers

- Oral sores

Note: The eye, nose, and mouth sensory points are located at an equal distance between the inferior border of the basic A zone and the middle border of the basic E zone on the Yin and Yang aspects of the scalp.

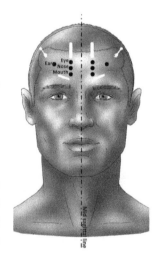

FIGURE 3.21

Ear point

Yin aspect: The point is located at the height of the upper third of the forehead and approximately 3.5 cm lateral to the mid-sagittal line (see Figures 3.22, 3.23, and 3.24).

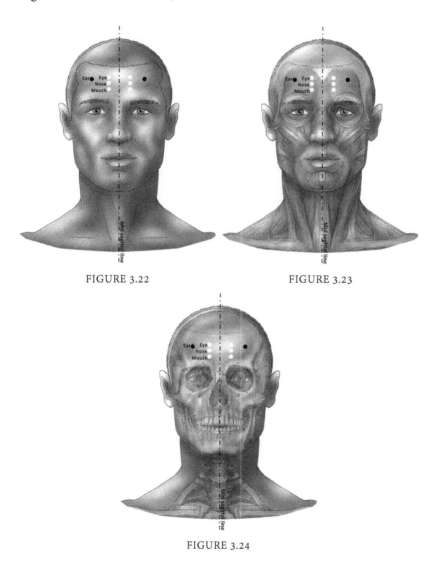

FIGURE 3.22   FIGURE 3.23

FIGURE 3.24

Yang aspect: The point is located at the height of the upper third of the occipital bone and approximately 2.5 cm lateral to the mid-sagittal line (see Figure 3.25).

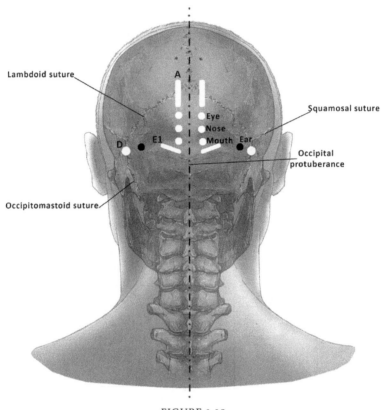

FIGURE 3.25

Yin and Yang indications:

- Tinnitus
- Fluid buildup in the ear (otitis media)
- Inflammation and infections of the ear
- Sudden deafness
- Auricular pain
- Loss of balance

Note: The ear point is located approximately 1 cm inferior to the basic C point at a 45° angle between the inferior border of the basic C point and 1 cm inferior to the nasal bridge.

Extrasensory points

As well as these four points, three additional points have been discovered: the throat, oral, and temporomandibular joint (TMJ) points. Three of the basic points can also be considered sensory points because needling these points also affects the sensory organs of the head (see Figure 3.26).

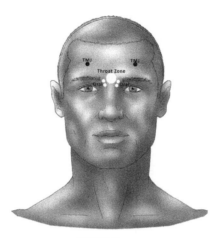

FIGURE 3.26

The throat, oral, and TMJ points are not located on the Yang aspect of the scalp. The oral and teeth points are needled to treat disorders of the mouth and teeth. The throat point is needled to treat any disorders of the throat region, and also the organs in the throat, such as the thyroid and parathyroid glands. The TMJ point is needled to treat any disorders of the TMJ.

All of the sensory points can be needled when there is a motor disorder of the muscles surrounding the sensory organ. For example, needling the eye point will affect the orbit muscle, and needling the nose point will affect activity of the alae nasi muscle. When this muscle is paralyzed, the practitioner can needle the nose and eye points to treat the paralysis.

Several sensory points can be needled concomitantly for treating some disorders. For example, concomitant needling of the nose, mouth, throat, and sometimes the ear point is often done when treating sinusitis, rhinitis, or any nasal obstruction. In this instance, the purpose of this concomitant needling is to increase the ability of the sinuses to drain the accumulated fluids.

Concomitant needling is also done when treating a patient with Bell's palsy (needle the sensory points and cranial nerve VII point concomitantly) or for trigeminal neuralgia (needle the sensory points and cranial nerve V point on the side on which the symptoms are present).

Concomitant needling can be done in a patient with impaired proprioception, which manifests itself as a lack of feeling on one side, a lack of acknowledgment of one side of the body, and sometimes dizziness or vertigo and instability. For such a patient, concomitant needling of the eye, ear, and cranial nerve VIII point can be done.

Concomitant needling can be done in a patient with hemispatial neglect of one side of the body, which usually occurs after a traumatic brain injury or a stroke. The symptoms of hemispatial neglect are lack of acknowledgment of any stimulation that originates from one side of the body. For example, a patient with right-side traumatic brain injury will not acknowledge any information that originates from the left side of the body. For such patients, concomitant needling of the four tinnitus points and the basic H point on the same side as the patient's hemispatial neglect can be done.

In general, when treating a patient with a disorder of the sensory organs, I always recommend needling the basic A point because needling this point also affects the head and the face in a general manner.

The oral and teeth, throat, and TMJ points are a second group of points that can also be needled for treating the sensory organs. The oral and teeth points will treat any disorders of the mouth and teeth. The throat point will treat any disorders of the throat region and also the organs near the throat, such as the thyroid and parathyroid glands. The TMJ point will treat disorders of the TMJ such as pain, bronchitis, temporal headaches and Bell's palsy.

The oral and teeth points also have a diagnostic zone. For a patient who complains of toothache, the patient's pain may originate from the opposite side. Accordingly, it is necessary to palpate the diagnostic area of the teeth and oral points, which are located on the medial aspect of the sternoclavicular joint (SCJ). The sensitivity of the side will determine which side will be needled.

Needling the oral and teeth points is also very effective for treating shoulder disorders for two reasons. First, the oral points also affect the hyoid bone and hyoid muscle, which connects to the acromion in the back region of the shoulder. When the oral and teeth points are needled, any tension in the hyoid muscle is released, and this will result in relaxing the shoulder. Second, there is a microsystem, the nasal microsystem, in which the whole body is reflected in the nose. In this microsystem, the medial orbits of the eyes are representations of the shoulder region (see Figure 3.27).

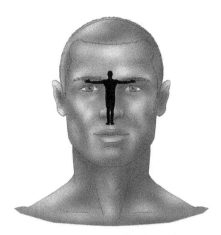

FIGURE 3.27

For treating a shoulder disorder, the points on the same side on which the symptom occurs are needled. If the patient complains of a right shoulder disorder, the right oral teeth point is needled.

The four-point needling combination for treating tinnitus

Tinnitus is the perception of noise or ringing in the ears when no sound is present and is a symptom of an underlying condition. There are two kinds of tinnitus: subjective tinnitus, which is caused by problems of the auditory nerves or auditory pathways in the brain, and objective tinnitus, which can be caused by orthopedic injuries or abnormal fluid pressure in the inner ear. The difference between the two types is that the tinnitus in objective tinnitus can sometimes last for an hour or two and then disappears.

Subjective tinnitus, which is usually a high-pitched or a low sound like a cricket or the ocean, is difficult to treat because it is due to nerve damage in the inner ear. Patients with subjective tinnitus should be referred to a physician or neurologist for treatment. If acupuncture is used to treat the patient, the high-pitched sound can be converted to a low-pitched sound, but very rarely will it disappear—treatment may result in its disappearance for several days, but the tinnitus will return.

Objective tinnitus can be caused by any orthopedic disorder in the neck, jaw, or mouth region. The treatment of objective tinnitus or any other ear disorder, such as pain, congestion, fluid in the ear, and sudden deafness, is a four-point needling combination that also affects and sharpens the vision. This comprises two Yin and Yang ear points (the Yin sensory ear point and Yang sensory ear point) that are located around the occipital bone, and two points, called Tinnitus 1 and Tinnitus 2, which are located on the Yin and Yang aspects of the scalp. The two Tinnitus points are located in bone divots on the upper borders of the temporalis muscle on an arch between the Yin and Yang ear points (see Figures 3.28, 3.29, and 3.30).

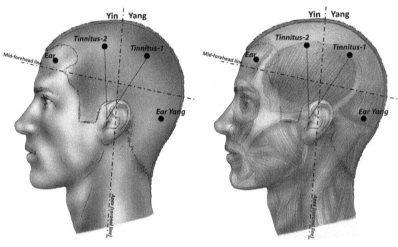

FIGURE 3.28   FIGURE 3.29

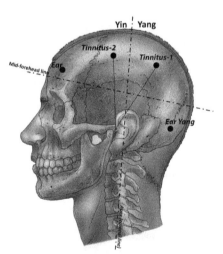

FIGURE 3.30

The Tinnitus 1 point is located approximately 4 cm above the apex of the ear and approximately 2–3 cm posterior to the apex line. The Tinnitus 2 point is located approximately 4 cm above the apex of the ear and approximately 3–4 cm anterior to the apex line.

Note: Both points are located on the superior borders of the temporalis muscle.

Needling these four points (the Yin and Yang ear points and the Tinnitus 1 and Tinnitus 2 points) is mandatory for treating objective tinnitus, and very often the tinnitus will go away and not return after treatment. When treating objective tinnitus, the practitioner can also include needling the basic A, B, and E points in the treatment.

Note: The four-point needling combination is also very effective for treating other neurological disorders, such as imbalance, hemispatial neglect syndrome, vertigo, and instability.

Brain and Spine Diagnostic Zones

Diagnostic Zones of the Basic and Brain Points

• • • • • •

The selection of a basic or brain point to needle is done by elbow or neck diagnosis (the latter will be discussed later). For elbow diagnosis, there are six diagnostic zones around the elbow and on the biceps muscle: three are located in the cubical fossa of the elbow, and three are located on the biceps muscle. Selection of the points to needle depends on the sensitivity of a diagnostic zone in the elbow and on the biceps muscle. For determining the side of the scalp that will be needled, selection is done according to the sensitivity of the side of the scalp. The points are needled ipsilateral to the diagnostic zone in the elbow.

Location of each diagnostic zone in elbow diagnosis

- The diagnostic zone for the neck (cervical) region is located between the lateral epicondyle and the LI-11 acupuncture point.

- The diagnostic zone for the thoracic region is located distal to the LU-5 acupuncture point.

- The diagnostic zone for the lumbar region is located between the medial epicondyle and the HT-3 acupuncture point.

- The diagnostic zone for the basal ganglia is located about 3 cm superior to the elbow in the center of the biceps muscle between the long head and short head of the biceps femoris muscle.

- The diagnostic zone for the cerebrum is located on the same line as that of the basal ganglia, but on the medial side of the short head of the biceps femoris muscle between the short head of the biceps femoris muscle and the brachialis muscle.

- The diagnostic zone for the cerebellum is located on the same line as that of the basal ganglia, but on the lateral side of the long head of the biceps femoris muscle between the long head of the biceps femoris muscle and the brachialis muscle.

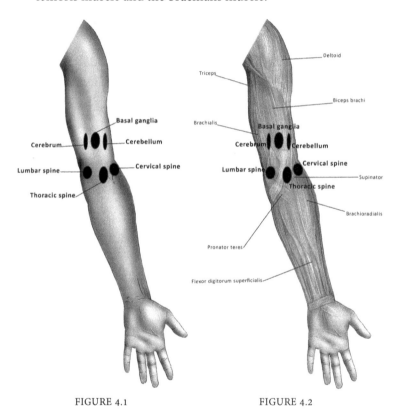

FIGURE 4.1   FIGURE 4.2

Using the basic and brain points for diagnosis and treatment

The best way for the practitioner to know that he or she has chosen the correct treatment is to repeatedly check the color of the palms of the patient's hand. One aim of the treatment is to obtain identical flow of qi and blood on both sides of the body. Once the practitioner has achieved this aim, the needles that have been inserted into the scalp can be withdrawn. Another aim is to achieve the same sensitivity of the LI-4 acupuncture point (abductor pollicis brevis muscle) in both hands. Once the practitioner has achieved this aim, it is not necessary to needle any additional points. The basic point protocol for using the elbow and basic points to treat a root and symptom is as follows:

- Examine and compare the palms of the hand to check for a good flow of qi and blood.

- Compare the responses to palpation of the LI-4 acupuncture point on both hands.

- The diagnostic zone in the elbow determines which side will be treated and which basic or brain point will be needled. Indicate if ipsilateral or contralateral.

- After needling, check whether sensitivity in the diagnostic zone is lessened.

- Check the sensitivity of the LI-4 acupuncture point to verify that sensitivity on both sides is the same.

- Check the blood flow and qi in both palms to verify that the palms of the hands have the same color.

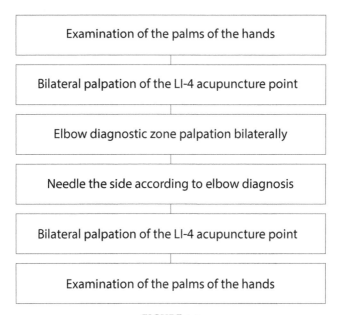

FIGURE 4.3

For example, a patient complains of right-sided neck pain:

- Examination of the palms of both hands reveals that the left palm is less vital than the right palm.

- Palpation of the LI-4 acupuncture point on the left and right sides of the hands reveals that the left side is more sensitive than the right side.

- After comparing the sensitivity of the diagnostic zones in the left and right elbow, the points that are most suitable for needling are the A point on the left side and the D point on the right side.

- After needling these two points, the responses to palpation of the LI-4 acupuncture point on the left and right sides are compared in order to check whether the sensitivity is the same on both sides and that sensitivity has lessened.

When starting treatment, the patient's spinal equilibrium also needs to be considered. According to the elbow diagnosis, the basic points A, D, E, F, and I will be the first points that are needled. If there is no improvement in the patient's symptoms after needling these points, the B, C, G, and H points are added to the needling regime.

Diagnostic zone	Needling point
Brain zones	Cerebral, cerebellum, basal ganglia
Cervical area	A, B, I
Thoracic area	E, I
Lumbar area	D, extra D, I, F, H

5

The Ypsilon (Internal Organ and Channel) Points

• • • • • • •

The Ypsilon points are a constellation of points that are located bilaterally on the temporal area of the scalp and form a somatotope of the 12 internal organs. The Ypsilon needling points on the Yin aspect are located in a rectangular area whose borders are the front hairline (anterior border), zygomatic arch (inferior border), mid-forehead (superior border), and ear apex (posterior border). The Ypsilon needling points are mirror-reflected in an area on the Yang aspect of the scalp at a 15° angle below the Ypsilon points on the Yin aspect of the scalp, whose borders are the apex line (anterior border), mastoid process (inferior border), mid-forehead (superior border), and occipitomastoid suture (posterior border) (see Figure 5.3).

The Ypsilon needling points are found at four different locations. The first and most used location is called strong Yin, and the second location is called strong Yang. The other two locations, which are rarely used, are called weak Yin and weak Yang. The points in the weak group are located in an area that is mirror-reflected above the strong group (see Figures 5.1 and 5.2).

Needling the Ypsilon points is mostly done to treat internal diseases, to strengthen the function of the internal organs, and to treat the entire length of the Chinese acupuncture channels (meridians) (see Figure 1.15).

Many disorders can be treated by needling the Ypsilon points, some of which are listed under the indications of the target organ. However, selecting a specific Ypsilon point to needle is determined by the resulting sensitivity of the diagnostic zone in the neck or abdomen, and not by the symptoms (see the explanation in the section on neck and abdomen diagnostic zones in Chapter 7).

Note: The same indications presented in this chapter of the Ypsilon needling points apply to the four groups (strong Yin and weak Yin, strong Yang and weak Yang) of the Ypsilon needling points.

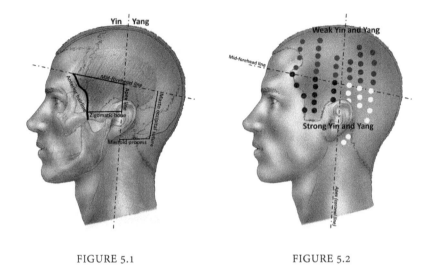

FIGURE 5.1   FIGURE 5.2

Locations and indications of the Ypsilon points
Yin aspect location

The following four points, the LU, SI, SJ, and LI points, are located near the anterior border on the front edge of the sideburn:

The **LU (Lung) point** is located where the front hairline and mid-forehead line meet.

Indications for needling:

- Chest pain
- Dyspnea
- Hyperventilation
- Asthma
- Bronchitis
- Disorders of the parathyroid gland

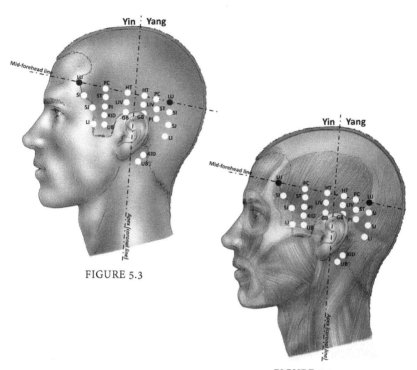

FIGURE 5.3

FIGURE 5.4

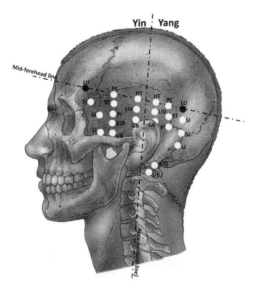

FIGURE 5.5

Lung channel

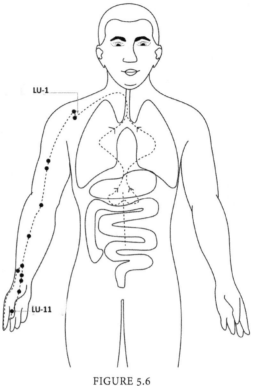

LU-1

LU-11

FIGURE 5.6

The **SI (Small Intestine) point** is located on the front hairline about 1 cm below the LU point.

Indications for needling:

- Bowel irregularities
- Crohn's disease
- Diarrhea
- Vomiting
- Lower abdomen pain
- Diverticulitis

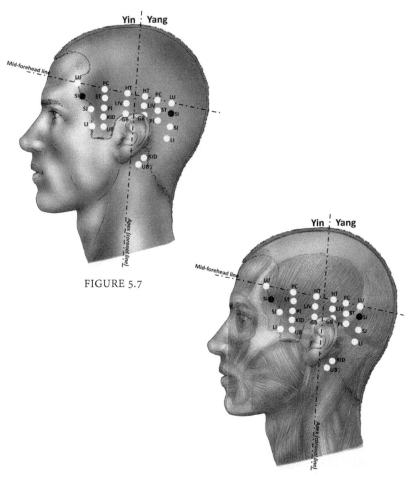

FIGURE 5.7

FIGURE 5.8

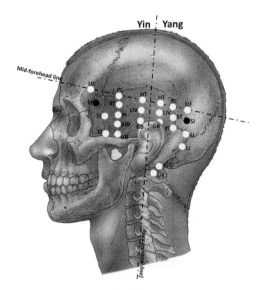

FIGURE 5.9

Small Intestine channel

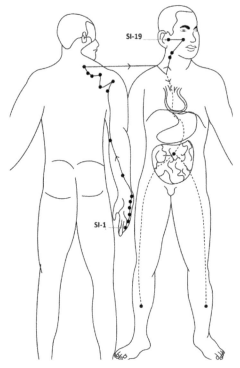

FIGURE 5.10

The **SJ (San Jiao) point** is located on the front hairline about 0.5 cm above the basic D point, which is about 1.5 cm above the zygomatic arch.

Indications for needling:

- High sugar levels in the body
- Immune disorders
- Gastric pain

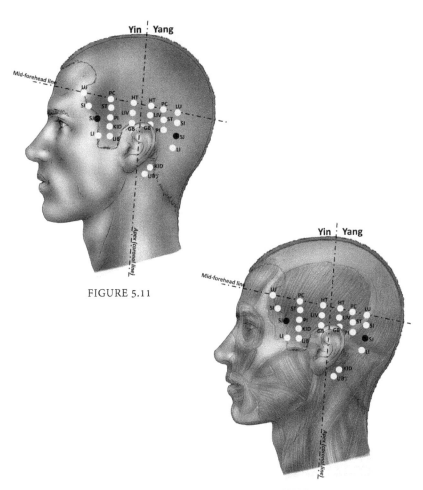

FIGURE 5.11

FIGURE 5.12

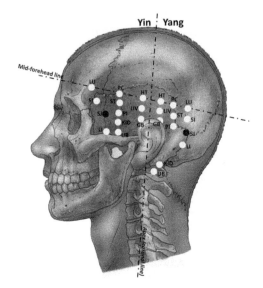

FIGURE 5.13

San Jiao channel

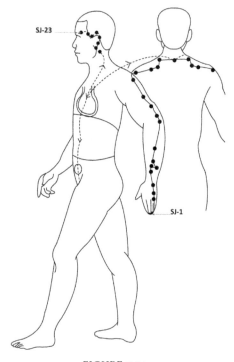

FIGURE 5.14

The **LI (Large Intestine) point** is located on the front hairline just above the zygomatic arch.

Indications for needling:

- Diarrhea
- Constipation
- Peptic ulcer
- Colitis

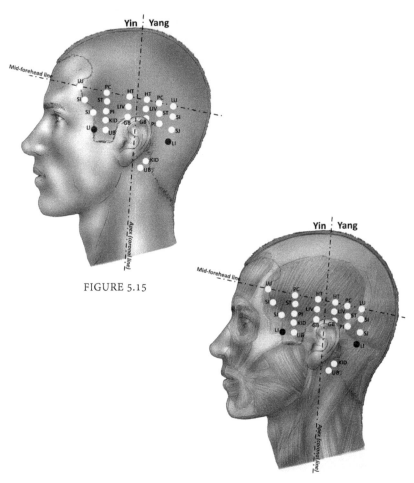

FIGURE 5.15

FIGURE 5.16

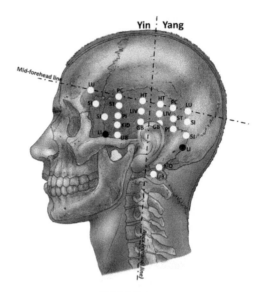

FIGURE 5.17

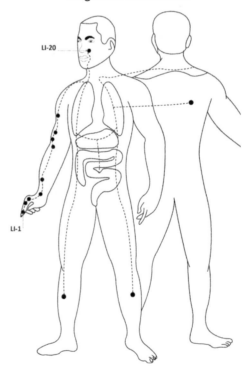

FIGURE 5.18

The following three points, the GB, HT, and LIV points, are located near the posterior border:

The **GB (Gallbladder) point** is located at the root of the ear, slightly anterior to the apex line.

Indications for needling:

- Cholecystitis
- Cholelithiasis

- Dyspepsia
- Swallowing disorders

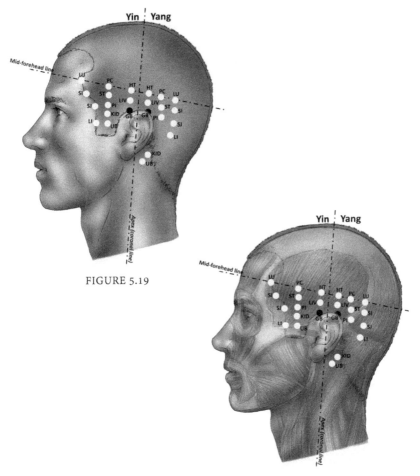

FIGURE 5.19

FIGURE 5.20

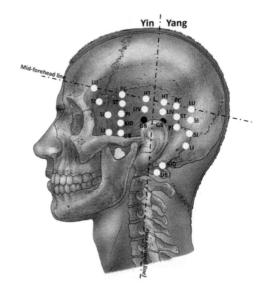

FIGURE 5.21

Gallbladder channel

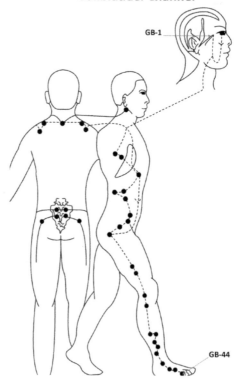

FIGURE 5.22

The **HT (Heart) point** is located approximately 3 cm above the root of the ear.

Indications for needling:

- Emotional stress
- Depression
- Angina pectoris
- Cardiac arrhythmia
- Tachycardia

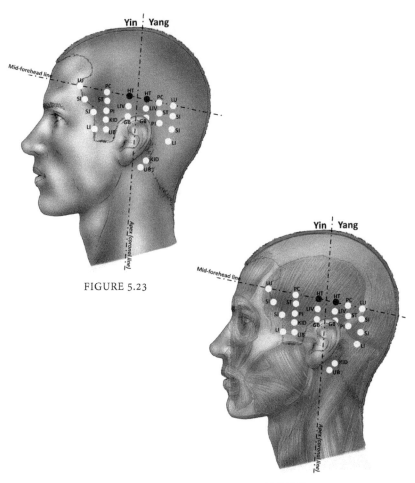

FIGURE 5.23

FIGURE 5.24

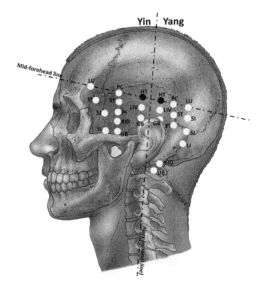

FIGURE 5.25

Heart channel

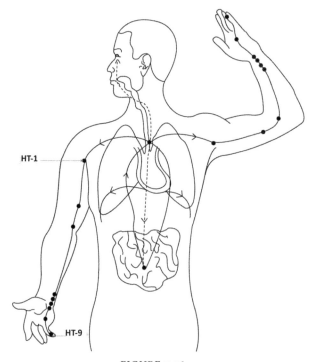

FIGURE 5.26

The **LIV (Liver) point** is located between the GB and HT points.

Indications for needling:

- Physical and emotional stress
- Hepatitis

- Headaches
- Migraine
- Insomnia

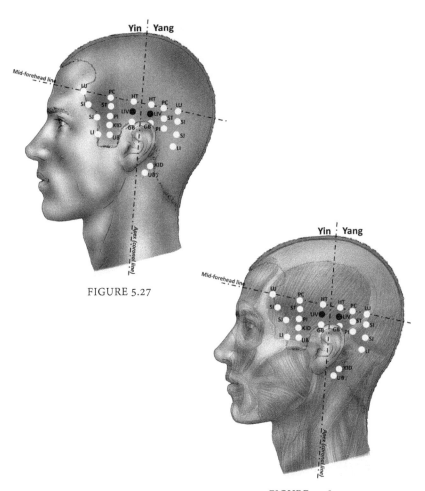

FIGURE 5.27

FIGURE 5.28

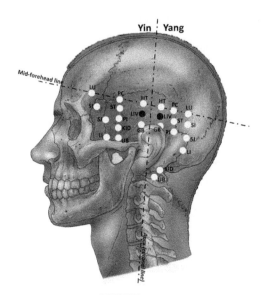

FIGURE 5.29

Liver channel

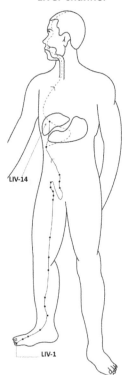

FIGURE 5.30

The following five points, the PC, ST, PI, UB, and KID points, are located between the front hairline and the apex line:

The **PC (Pericardium) point** is located between the HT and LU points.

Indications for needling:

- Physical stress
- Depression
- Angina pectoris
- Cardiac arrhythmia
- Tachycardia

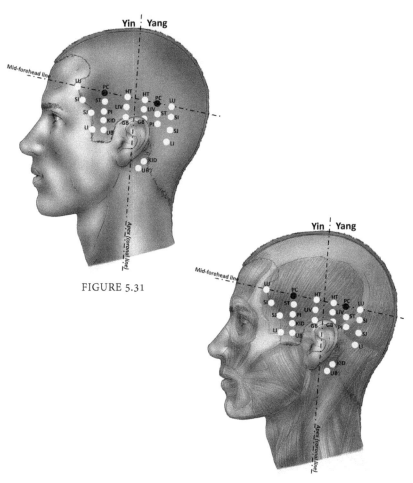

FIGURE 5.31

FIGURE 5.32

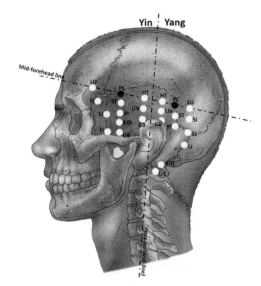

FIGURE 5.33

Pericardium channel

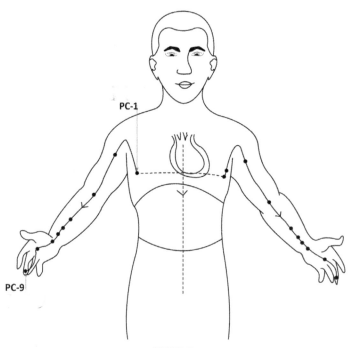

FIGURE 5.34

The **ST (Stomach) point** is located between the SI and LIV points.

Indications for needling:

- Gastritis
- Stomach ulcers
- Trigeminal neuralgia
- Digestive disturbances

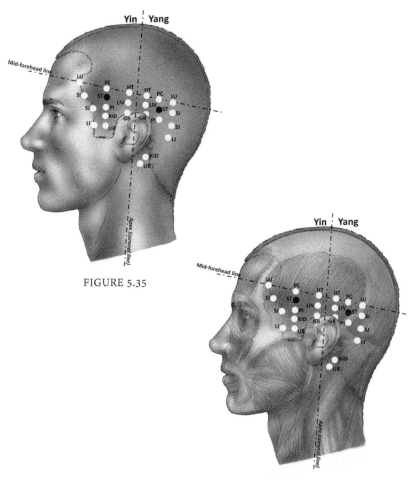

FIGURE 5.35

FIGURE 5.36

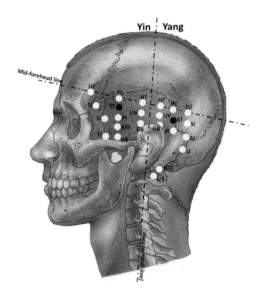

FIGURE 5.37

Stomach chanel

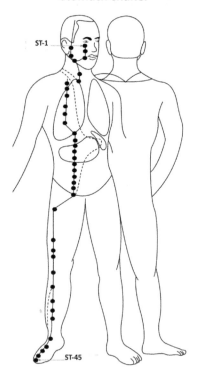

FIGURE 5.38

The **PI (Spleen/Pancreas) point** is located between the SJ and GB points.

Indications for needling:

- Diabetes
- Pancreatitis

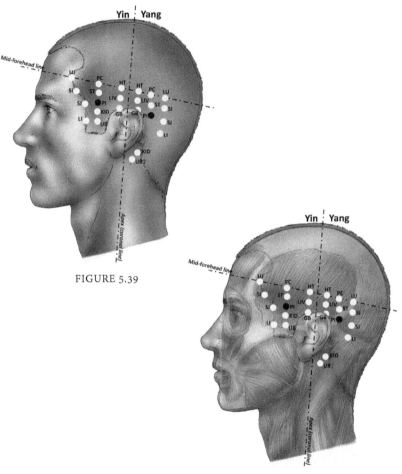

FIGURE 5.39

FIGURE 5.40

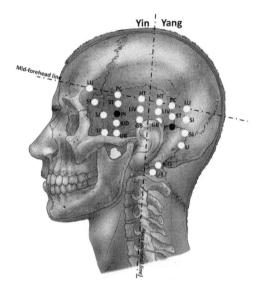

FIGURE 5.41

Pl/Spleen channel

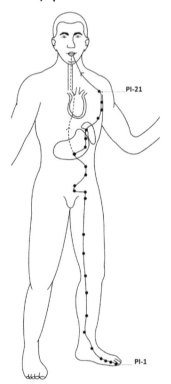

FIGURE 5.42

The **UB (Urinary Bladder) point** is located in the center of the sideburn, just above the zygomatic arch.

Indications for needling:

- Renal disorders
- Calculus
- Polyuria
- Urine retention
- Prostatic hypertrophy

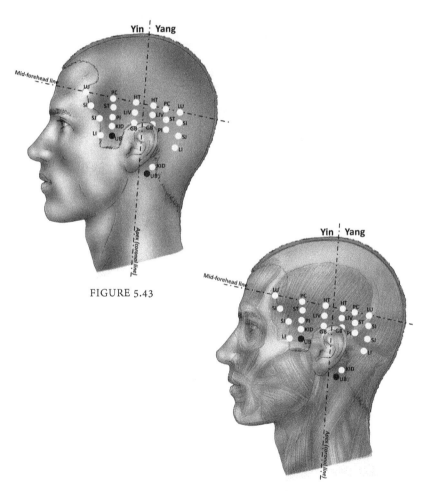

FIGURE 5.43

FIGURE 5.44

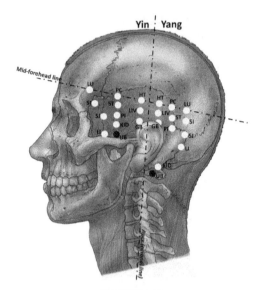

FIGURE 5.45

Urinary Bladder channel

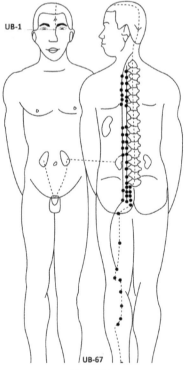

FIGURE 5.46

The **KID (Kidney) point** is located between the PI and UB points.

Indications for needling:

- Kidney stones
- Multiple sclerosis
- Fibromyalgia
- Hemiplegia
- Knee and skin disorders

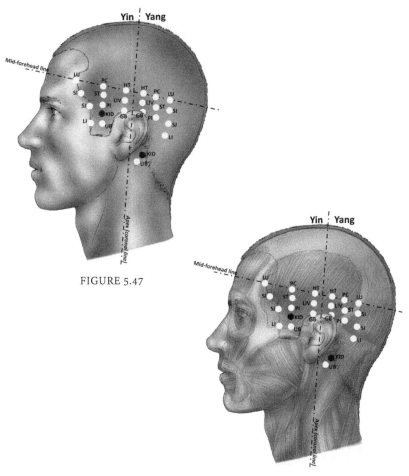

FIGURE 5.47

FIGURE 5.48

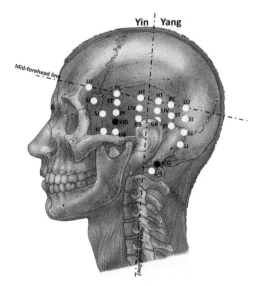

FIGURE 5.49

Kidney channel

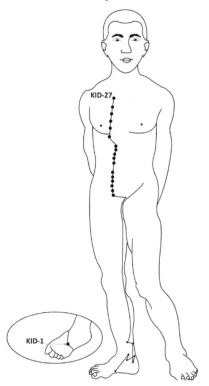

FIGURE 5.50

Yang aspect location

The following four points, the LU, SI, SJ, and LI points, are located on the occipitomastoid suture and lambdoid suture:

The **LU point** is located where the lambdoid suture and the mid-forehead line meet.

The **SI point** is located on the lambdoid suture about 1 cm below the LU point.

The **SJ point** is located on the occipitomastoid suture about 0.5 cm above the basic D point on the Yang aspect.

The **LI point** is located on the occipitomastoid suture, approximately 0.5 cm below the basic D point on the Yang aspect.

The following three points, the GB, HT, and LIV points, are located near the apex line:

The **GB point** is located at the height of the root of the ear and slightly posterior to the apex line or the superior auricular muscle.

The **HT point** is located where the GB point and mid-forehead line meet.

The **LIV point** is located between the GB and HT points.

The following three points, the PC, ST, and PI points, are located between the occipitomastoid suture and the apex line:

The **PC point** is located between the HT and LU points.

The **ST point** is located between the SI and LIV points.

The **PI point** is located between the SJ and GB points.

The following two points, the KID and UB points, are located around the mastoid process:

The **KID point** is located in a small notch on the posterior border of the mastoid process.

The **UB point** is located approximately 1 cm below the Ypsilon KID point on the sternocleidomastoid muscle (SCM) on the Yang aspect.

Needling these points requires a greater understanding than that required for needling the basic, brain, and sensory points because of their inherent complex function. In addition to exerting an effect on the internal organs, needling these points also exerts an effect on other systems according to traditional Chinese medicine. Additionally, needling these points exerts a wide-ranging effect that is greater than that observed after needling the basic, brain, and sensory points. For example, needling the LIV point will affect the liver and liver function. Needling this point will balance the internal systems of the body, will improve sleep, and relieve shoulder pain that is caused by supraspinatus muscle tension. Therefore, the greater the knowledge and understanding of traditional Chinese medicine, the better the ability to use these points. The exact mechanism of the action after needling these points is yet to be fully understood.

6

Cranial Nerve Points

• • • • • •

There are 12 pairs of cranial nerves that emerge from the brain and innervate the head, face, neck, chest, heart, and digestive tract. Cranial nerves 1 and 2 emerge from the brain, and cranial nerves 3–12 emerge from the brain stem. Dr Yamamoto found a link between each cranial nerve point and a particular meridian. An abdominal or neck diagnosis is required for selecting the correct needling point(s).

The functions of the cranial nerve points are the same as those of the Ypsilon points. In addition, needling a cranial nerve point can exert an effect on that cranial nerve. Needling the cranial nerve points exerts an effect on the central nervous system, whereas needling the Ypsilon points exerts an effect on the peripheral nervous system. For a patient with a disorder with a specific cranial nerve, it is better to needle the cranial nerve points and not the Ypsilon points. For example, trigeminal neuralgia is a chronic pain condition that affects cranial nerve 5 (the trigeminal nerve) that innervates the ST organ (according to traditional Chinese medicine) and innervates the facial mucosa and skin and conveys sensory information from contact of a stimulus with the facial skin or the face's mucosa (according to western medical science). Therefore, it is better to needle the cranial nerve point on the scalp than to needle the ST Ypsilon point. It is also important to know the functions of each cranial nerve in order to needle the correct cranial nerve when it is not functioning and to know which organ is associated with each cranial nerve (see the table at the end of the chapter).

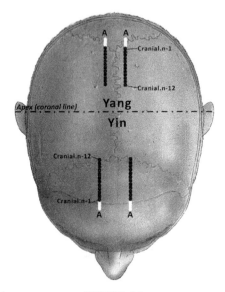

FIGURE 6.1

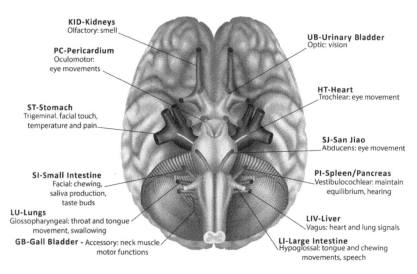

FIGURE 6.2

Location of the cranial nerve points
Yin aspect location

The 12 cranial nerve points are located on a 6–8 cm vertical line directly above the superior region of the basic A needling point and the frontal suture. The distance between each needling point is approximately

0.5 cm. The first four cranial nerve needling points are located above the superior region of the basic A point. Cranial nerves 1, 2, 3, and 4, that are associated with the Kidney, Urinary Bladder, Pericardium, and Heart organs, respectively (according to the YNSA microsystem), overlap the cerebral zone (the same needling points).

The 5th and 6th cranial nerve needling points (cranial nerves 5 and 6), that are associated with the Stomach and San Jiao organs, respectively (according to the YNSA microsystem), overlap the cerebellar zone (the same needling points).

The 12th cranial nerve point is located on the coronal suture.

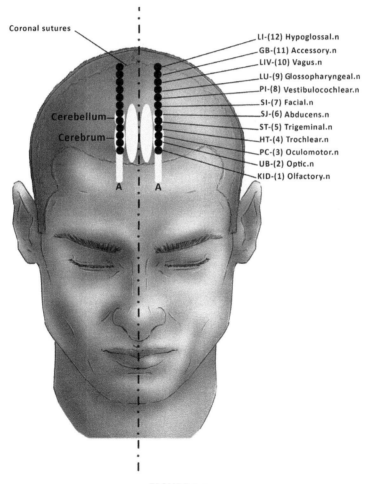

FIGURE 6.3

Yang aspect location

These 12 cranial nerve points are located directly above the basic A point on a vertical line that is approximately 5–6 cm. The distance between each needling point is approximately 0.5 cm. The needling point of the first cranial nerve Yang point is located close to the basic A Yang point. The needling point of the 12th cranial nerve point is located approximately 5–6 cm anterior to the superior region of the basic A Yang needling point.

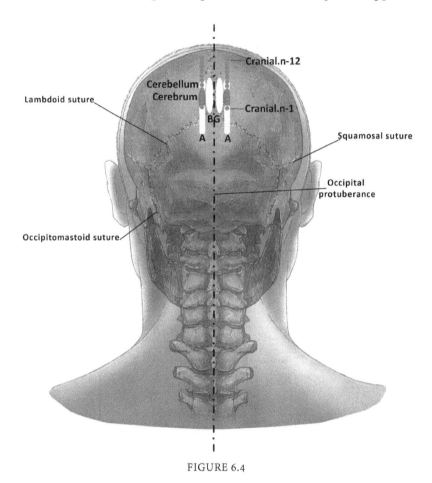

FIGURE 6.4

Cranial nerve number	Chinese medicine organ and channel association with the cranial nerve	Latin name	Western medical science
1	Kidney (KID)	Olfactorius	The sensory nerve of smell
2	Urinary Bladder (UB)	Opticus	The nerve that transfers visual information to the vision centers of the brain
3	Pericardium (PC)	Oculomotorius	The nerve that innervates four of the six extra-ocular muscles that control movement of the eye
4	Heart (HT)	Trochlearius	The nerve that innervates the superior oblique muscle, which enables looking down and up and rotation in the plane of the face
5	Stomach (ST)	Trigeminus	The sensory nerve of the face
6	San Jiao (SJ)	Abduceus	The nerve that innervates the muscle that abducts the eye
7	Small Intestine (SI)	Facialis	The nerve that innervates the muscles of the face and salivary glands and transfers sensory information on taste from the anterior two-thirds of the tongue
8	Spleen/Pancreas (PI)	Vestibulocohlearis	The nerve that transfers information about hearing and balance from the ear to the brain

Cranial nerve number	Chinese medicine organ and channel association with the cranial nerve	Latin name	Western medical science
9	Lung (LU)	Glossopharyngeus	A sensory and motor nerve that innervates various structures in the head and neck. It is important in swallowing because it elevates the larynx during swallowing
10	Liver (LIV)	Vagus	The main nerve of the parasympathetic nervous system, and its functions are both motor and sensory
11	Gallbladder (GB)	Accessorius	A motor nerve that innervates the sternocleidomastoid and trapezius muscles
12	Large Intestine (LI)	Hypoglossus	A motor nerve that innervates almost all muscles of the tongue

7

Diagnostic Zones of the Ypsilon and Cranial Nerve Points

• • • • • •

Neck diagnostic zone

The sensitivity of and tension of the muscles in the neck diagnostic zone determine which Ypsilon or cranial nerve point will be needled. When sensitivity or tension is found in a specific neck diagnostic zone, the practitioner will needle the specific Ypsilon or cranial nerve point that is associated with that specific diagnostic zone in the abdomen or neck.

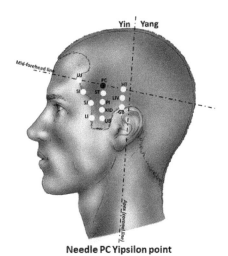

Needle PC Yipsilon point

FIGURE 7.1

For example, a 45-year-old man complains of left-side shoulder pain. Palpation of the Pericardium organ zone in the neck diagnostic zone on the left side reveals increased sensitivity of the zone. Accordingly, the PC Ypsilon needling point or the PC cranial nerve needling point on the left side will be needled.

Dr Yamamoto discovered the diagnostic zone in the neck several years after discovering the abdomen diagnostic zone. Nowadays, the neck diagnostic zone is more frequently used than the abdomen diagnostic zone. The neck diagnostic zone is a specific diagnostic zone in YNSA and differs from the abdomen diagnostic zone that was derived from traditional oriental medicine and was modified by Dr Yamamoto for the YNSA method.

How to palpate the neck diagnostic zone

The neck diagnostic test zone is palpated using the upper third of the thumb in the same way as one palpates the elbow diagnostic zone (see Chapter 4).

When palpating the neck, the practitioner's other hand will palpate the other side of the neck; when the practitioner is using the right thumb to palpate the neck, the practitioner's left thumb will palpate the right side of the neck and vice versa.

The pressure applied in the neck diagnosis should not exceed 750 grams (1.6 lbs). If you are unsure what 750 grams (1.6 lbs) of pressure feels like, I recommend applying the pressure to a scale to get the feeling of how much pressure it is.

The practitioner should needle the cranial nerve or Ypsilon point according to the most sensitive point in the diagnostic zones in the neck or abdomen.

Location and palpation of the neck diagnostic zone
Kidney (KID)

Location: The posterior division of the sternocleidomastoid muscle (SCM) and the clavicle.

Palpation and comments: Pressure is applied towards the scapula using the thumb.

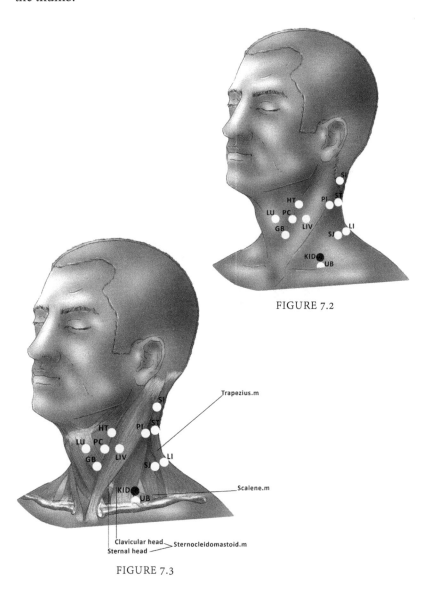

FIGURE 7.2

FIGURE 7.3

Urinary Bladder (UB)

Location: The same location as the Kidney diagnostic zone and partly behind the clavicle.

Palpation and comments: Pressure is applied downwards and posterior to the clavicle using the thumb.

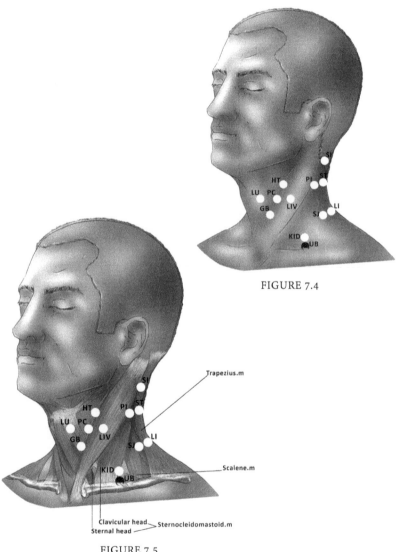

FIGURE 7.4

FIGURE 7.5

Liver (LIV)

Location: The center of the SCM at the level of the throat midway between the clavicle and the mandibular angle.

Palpation and comments: The thumb is moved back and forth across the SCM with a very gentle touch.

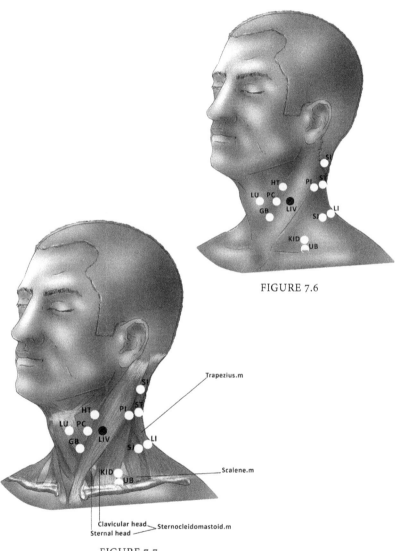

FIGURE 7.6

FIGURE 7.7

Pericardium (PC)

Location: The anterior division of the SCM at the level of the Liver diagnostic zone. The point is located on the anterior borders of the SCM.

Palpation and comments: Pressure is applied to the anterior border of the SCM in an anterior direction using the thumb.

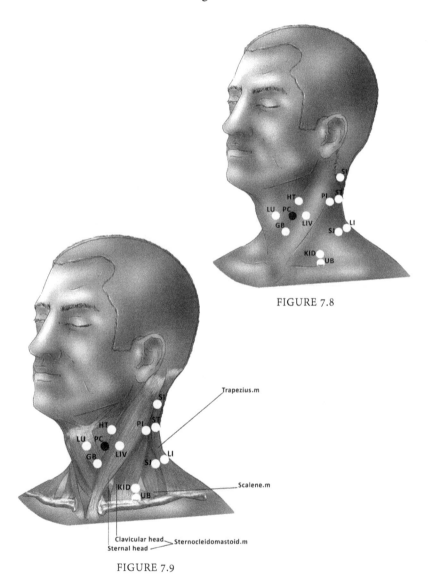

FIGURE 7.8

FIGURE 7.9

Heart (HT)

Location: The anterior border of the SCM at about a 45° angle above the Liver diagnostic zone. The point is located on the anterior borders of the SCM.

Palpation and comments: Pressure is applied at a 45° angle in an upward direction to the anterior border of the SCM using the thumb.

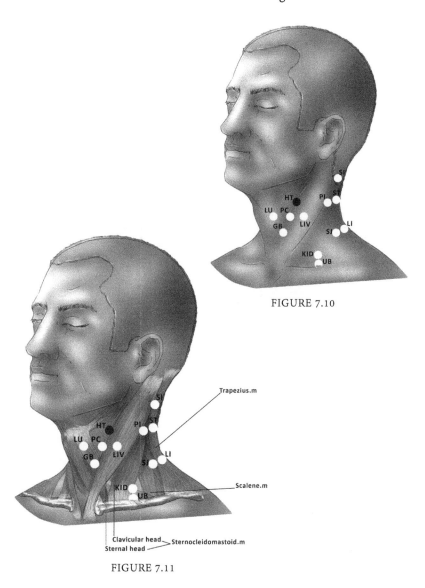

FIGURE 7.10

FIGURE 7.11

Gallbladder (GB)

Location: The anterior border of the SCM at about a 45° angle below the Liver diagnostic zone.

Palpation and comments: Pressure is applied at a 45° angle in a downward direction to the anterior border of the SCM using the thumb.

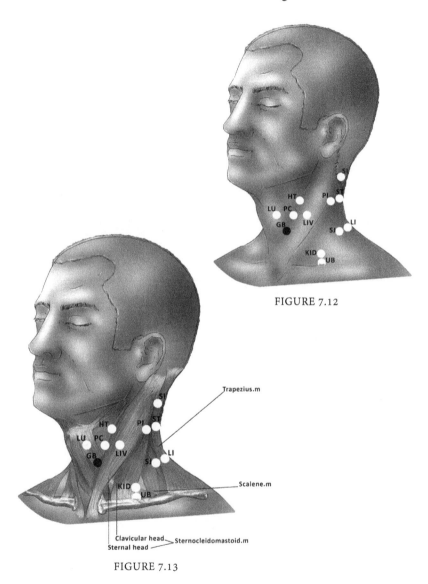

FIGURE 7.12

FIGURE 7.13

Small Intestine (SI)

Location: The meeting point of the mandibular angle and the anterior border of the trapezius muscle (in the area of the SJ-16 acupuncture point).

Palpation and comments: Light pressure is needed when palpating.

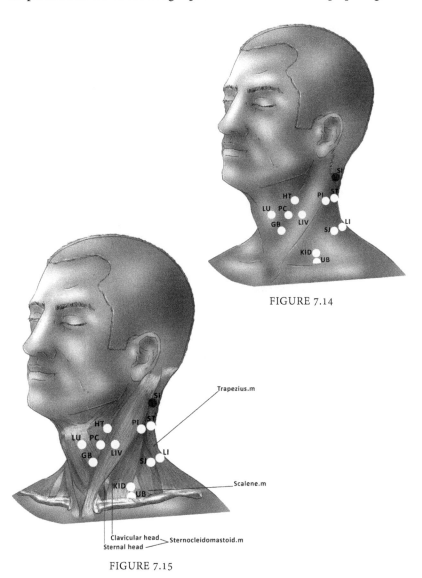

FIGURE 7.14

FIGURE 7.15

Stomach (ST)

Location: On the vertical division fibers of the trapezius muscle, at midway height between the Large Intestine neck diagnostic zone and the Small Intestine neck diagnostic zone. (This point is located at the same level as the Large Intestine neck diagnostic zone on the trapezius muscle.)

Palpation and comments: Light pressure is needed when palpating.

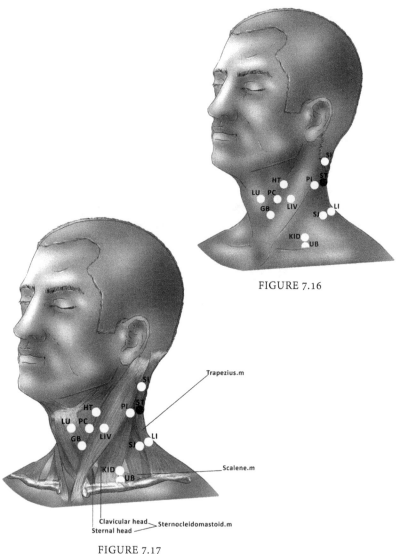

FIGURE 7.16

FIGURE 7.17

Spleen/Pancreas (Pl)

Location: Anterior to the vertical division fibers of the trapezius muscle, at midway between the Large Intestine and Small Intestine neck diagnostic zones. (This point is located at the same level as the Large Intestine neck diagnostic zone in the neck on the trapezius muscle.)

Palpation and comments: The thumb is moved from the Stomach diagnostic zone. The pressure can change from gentle to strong.

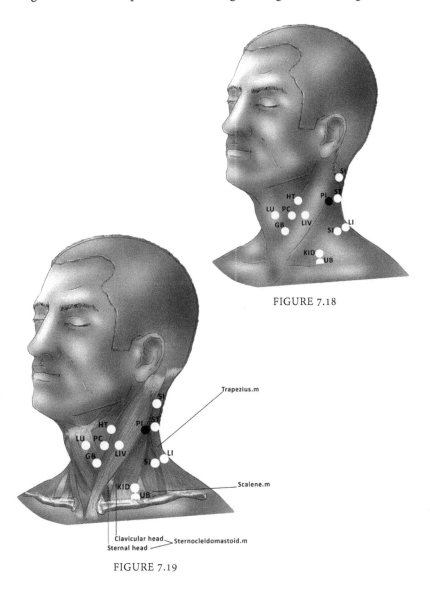

FIGURE 7.18

FIGURE 7.19

Large Intestine (LI)

Location: On the trapezius muscle where the horizontal division fibers and the upper trapezius muscle fibers merge (the area in the neck where the neck and shoulder meet) and slightly medial and slightly anterior to the GB-21 acupuncture point.

Palpation and comments: The thumb should roll on the muscle. Gentle pressure is needed.

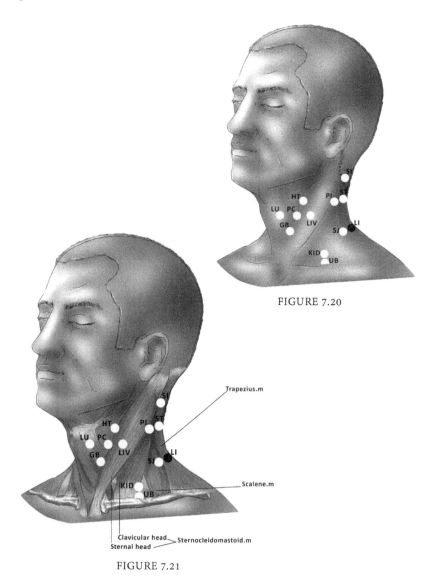

FIGURE 7.20

FIGURE 7.21

San Jiao (SJ)

Location: The anterior border of the trapezius muscle where the horizontal and vertical fibers of the trapezius muscle meet.

Palpation and comments: The thumb is moved from the Large Intestine diagnostic test zone anterior to the trapezius muscle.

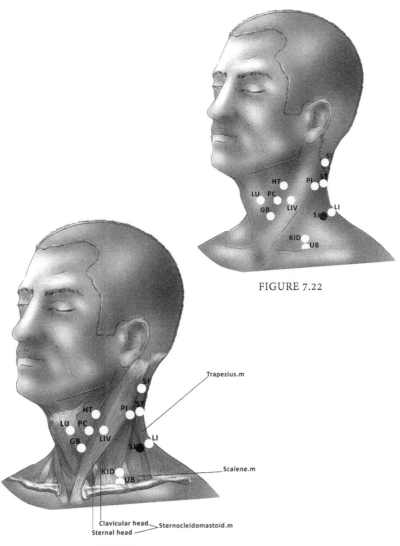

FIGURE 7.22

FIGURE 7.23

Lung (LU)

Location: Lateral to the thyroid cartilage.

Palpation and comments: Apply gentle pressure to both sides of the thyroid.

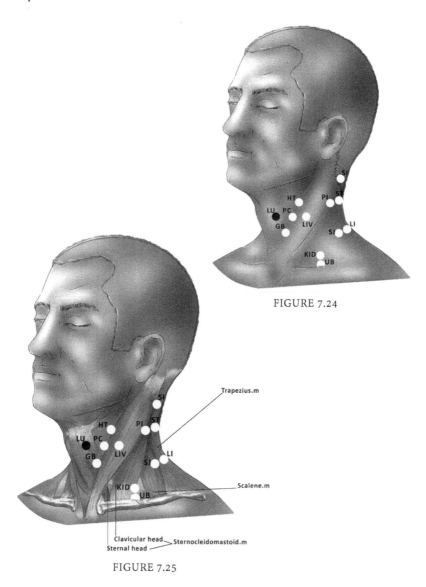

FIGURE 7.24

FIGURE 7.25

Abdomen diagnostic zone

Abdominal diagnosis was the first method that Dr Yamamoto used to diagnose internal problems and to select the Ypsilon or cranial needling points. Dr Yamamoto modified the method of abdominal diagnosis in traditional Chinese and Japanese medicine for diagnosing in YNSA. For this reason, there is considerable similarity between the two abdominal diagnostic maps of YNSA and Chinese and Japanese traditional medicines. Nowadays, abdominal diagnosis is less used than neck and elbow diagnoses, which were developed later. Since abdominal and neck diagnoses are associated with the Ypsilon and cranial nerve points, the practitioner should use the diagnostic method with which they feel more confident.

If the patient does not display sensitivity in the neck region, abdominal diagnosis is recommended, or if the patient does not display sensitivity when using abdominal diagnosis, then neck diagnosis is recommended.

As discussed in the section on neck diagnosis (see above), the choice of which Ypsilon or cranial nerve point to be needled is determined by the sensitivity of the equivalent organ zone when palpating the abdomen diagnostic zone.

The practitioner may feel tenderness, tightness, or softness, and increased sensitivity when palpating the abdomen diagnostic zone. When a practitioner finds one of these sensations in a specific diagnostic zone, it is an indication to needle the specific Ypsilon or cranial nerve needling point that is associated with the specific diagnostic zone in the abdomen.

When the practitioner finds sensitivity in one of the organ zones in the abdomen or neck diagnostic zone, the practitioner should needle the corresponding Ypsilon or cranial nerve point. After needling the point, the practitioner should again palpate the specific diagnostic zone to establish whether there is any change in sensitivity. If the correct Ypsilon or cranial nerve point has been needled, sensitivity in the diagnostic zone will wane.

The areas of the specific diagnostic zones of the Ypsilon or cranial nerve points in abdominal diagnosis are much larger and better defined than those in neck diagnosis.

In the abdomen diagnostic zone, there are zones for the brain, cervical spine, thoracic spine, and lumbar spine.

Location of the abdomen diagnostic zone
Abdomen diagnostic zones on the linea alba
HT = 1–2 cm below the xiphoid process.

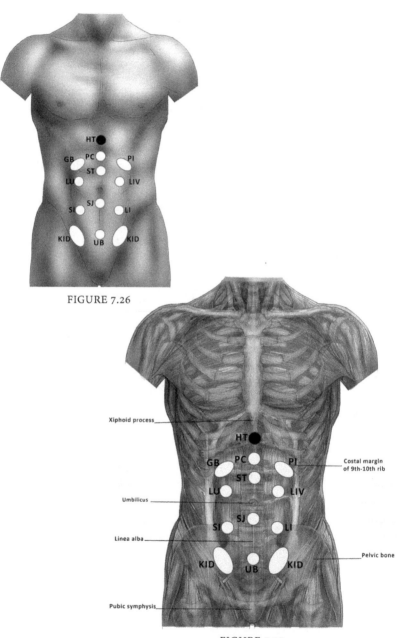

FIGURE 7.26

FIGURE 7.27

PC = 1–2 cm below the HT zone.

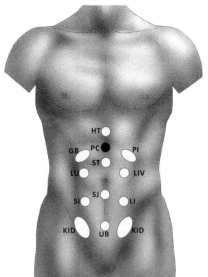

FIGURE 7.28

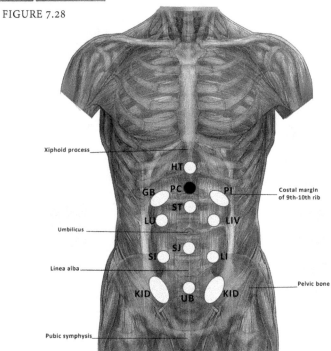

FIGURE 7.29

ST = 6–7 cm above the umbilicus or midway between the xiphoid process and the umbilicus.

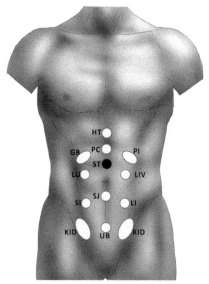

FIGURE 7.30

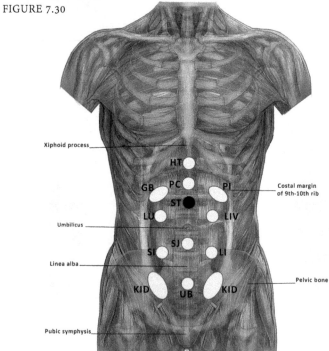

FIGURE 7.31

SJ = 2–3 cm below the umbilicus.

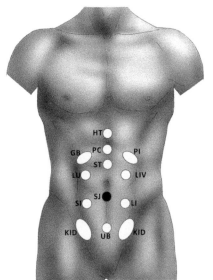

FIGURE 7.32

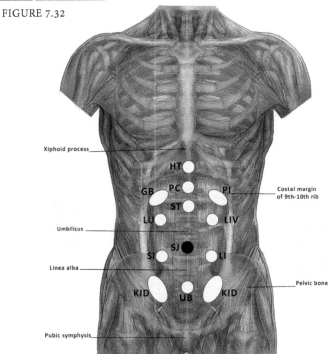

FIGURE 7.33

UB = 2–3 cm above the center of the pubic symphysis.

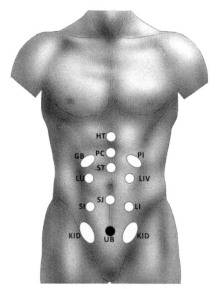

FIGURE 7.34

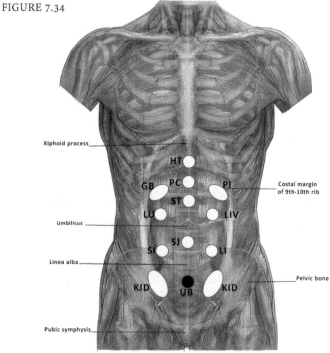

FIGURE 7.35

Diagnostic zones on the right side of the abdomen

GB = directly below the right costal margin.

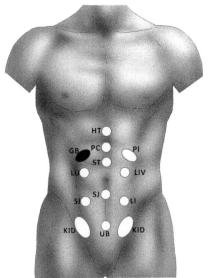

FIGURE 7.36

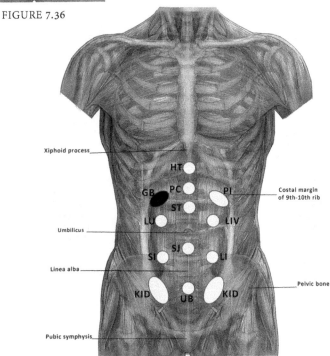

FIGURE 7.37

LU = on a 45° angle upward line from the umbilicus between the right costal margin and the umbilicus.

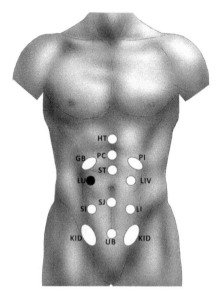

FIGURE 7.38

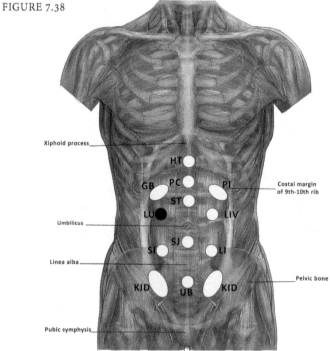

FIGURE 7.39

SI = approximately 6 cm from the right side of the umbilicus on a 45° angle downward line from the umbilicus.

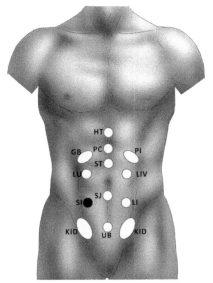

FIGURE 7.40

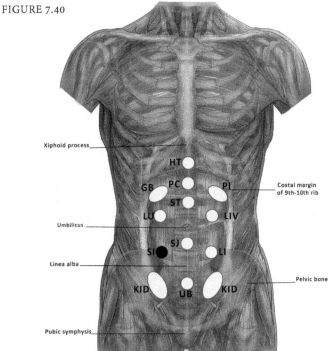

FIGURE 7.41

Diagnostic zones on the left side of the abdomen

PI = directly below the left costal margin.

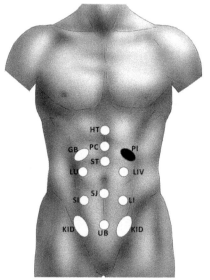

FIGURE 7.42

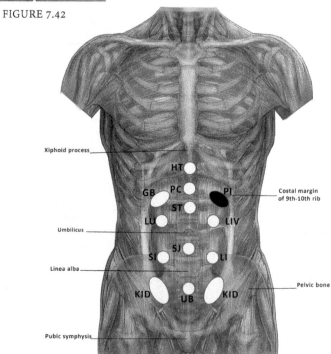

FIGURE 7.43

LIV = on a 45° angle upward line from the umbilicus between the left costal margin and the umbilicus.

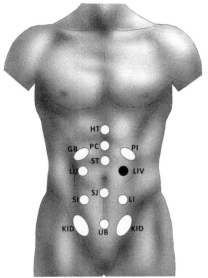

FIGURE 7.44

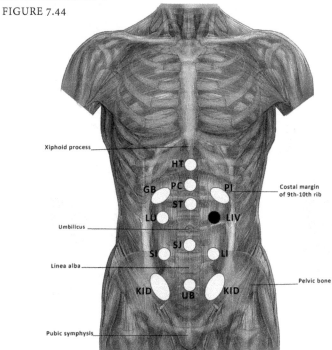

FIGURE 7.45

LI = on a 45° angle downward line from the umbilicus, approximately 6 cm from the left side of the umbilicus.

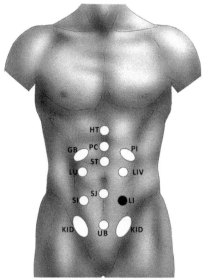

FIGURE 7.46

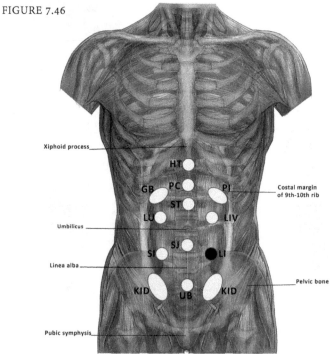

FIGURE 7.47

KID = bilaterally above the pelvic bone in the area of the GB-27 acupuncture point (the Kidney diagnostic zone is the only diagnostic zone that is located bilaterally).

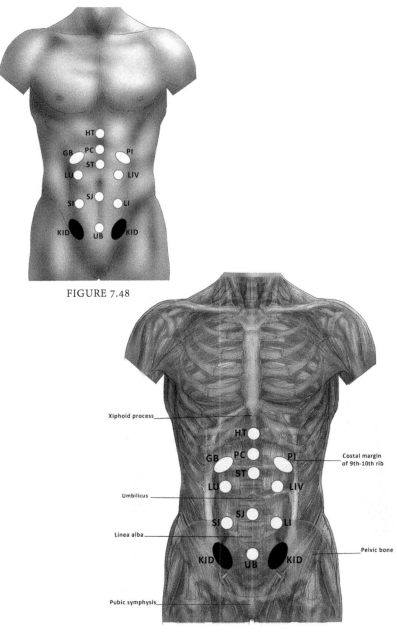

FIGURE 7.48

FIGURE 7.49

The three brain diagnostic zones are located on and around the xiphoid process (see Figure 7.50).

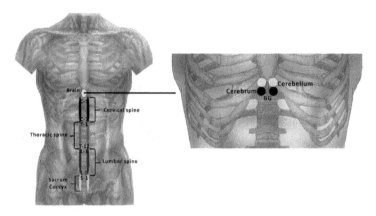

FIGURE 7.50

The basal ganglia diagnostic zone is located on the xiphoid process. When the basal ganglia diagnostic zone is found to be sensitive when palpated, the practitioner will needle the old basal ganglia needling zone (see Chapter 3 under the heading "Basal ganglia zone").

The cerebellum and cerebrum diagnostic zones are located on the superior aspect of the rectus abdominis muscle, lateral to the xiphoid process and medial to the costal cartilage of the seventh rib. These two zones are located bilaterally.

The cerebellum diagnostic zone is located in the upper corner of this area (on the rectus abdominis muscle, in the corner of the integration of the costal cartilage of the seventh rib and the xiphoid process).

The cerebrum diagnostic zone is located directly below the cerebellum diagnostic zone. This diagnostic zone is located on the RAM and lateral to the xiphoid process.

When the cerebellum or cerebrum diagnostic zones are sensitive when palpated by the practitioner, the specific zone will be needled (see Chapter 3 under the heading "Cerebral zone").

Spine diagnostic zone
Location of the spine diagnostic zone

The diagnostic zones of the cervical spine, thoracic spine, lumbar spine, and sacrum and coccyx are all located bilaterally on the lateral borders of the linea alba (KID acupuncture channel line).

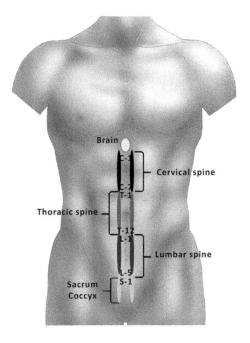

FIGURE 7.51

Cervical spine = The location of the diagnostic zone of the cervical spine (C1 vertebral region) begins approximately 1 cm below the xiphoid process and extends downward to approximately 7 cm below the xiphoid process (C7 vertebral region).

Thoracic spine = The location of the diagnostic zone of the thoracic spine begins 7 cm below the xiphoid process (T1 vertebral region) and extends downward to approximately 2 cm below the umbilicus (T12 vertebral region).

Lumbar spine = The location of the diagnostic zone of the lumbar spine begins approximately 2 cm below the umbilicus (L1 vertebral region) and extends downwards to approximately 3 cm above the pubic bone (L5 vertebral region).

Sacrum and coccyx = The location of the diagnostic zone of the sacrum and coccyx begins approximately 3 cm above the pubic bone (S1 region) and extends downwards to the inferior border of the pubic bone (coccyx egion).

Using the diagnostic zones for needling the Ypsilon or cranial nerve points

1. Examine and compare the palms of the hand to check the flow of qi and blood.

2. Compare the responses to palpation of the LI-4 acupuncture point on the right and left sides. The Ypsilon or cranial nerve points on the more sensitive side will be needled.

3. The response to palpation of the LI-4 point on the right and left sides are again compared after needling. If there is no sensitivity of the LI-4 acupuncture point, there is no need for any additional needling.

4. If there is no difference in response to palpation of the LI-4 acupuncture point on the right and left sides, the needles are kept in place for 30 minutes.

5. If the response to palpation of the LI-4 acupuncture point on the less sensitive side is greater than that of the more sensitive side, the Ypsilon or cranial nerve points of the less sensitive side are needled.

6. If the response to palpation of the LI-4 acupuncture point on the more sensitive side is still greater than that of the less sensitive side response, the basic points are needled according to the elbow diagnosis.

7. The protocol is repeated until there is no difference in response to palpation of the LI-4 acupuncture point on the right and left sides.

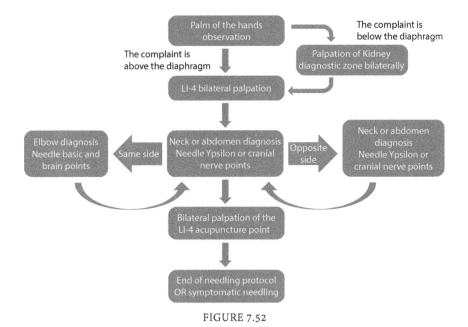

FIGURE 7.52

Note: When the patient's complaint involves an area below the diaphragm, the sensitivity of the Kidney diagnostic zone determines the side to be needled.

8

Additional Points and Somatotopes

• • • • • •

I somatotope

The I somatotope is a bilateral somatotope that is located in the ear region. It was recently developed from basic point I and contains an image of the entire body. This somatotope, which is needled to treat problems of the musculoskeletal system, has three areas:

- The **lower lumber** area extends along the mastoid bone and ascends to approximately 4–5 cm above the ear. The diagnostic zone for this is located in the area of the medial epicondyle (see Chapter 4).

- The **thoracic spine** area extends along the apex line and ascends to approximately 4–5 cm above the apex of the ear. The most superior part of this line corresponds to the area where thoracic vertebra 12 and lumbar vertebra 1 meet. The diagnostic zone for this area is the distal area of the LU-5 acupuncture point (see Chapter 4).

- The **upper cervical** area extends from the notch where the root of the ear merges with the face and extends to a height that is twice the length of the ear. The diagnostic zone for this area is the lateral epicondyle (see Chapter 4).

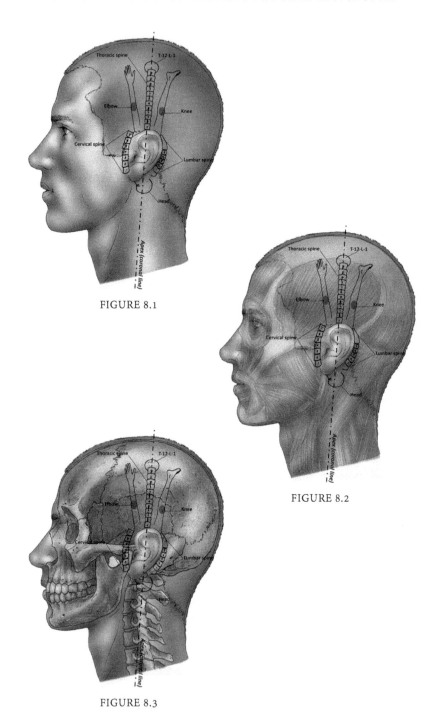

FIGURE 8.1

FIGURE 8.2

FIGURE 8.3

Master key points

The master key points are four needling points that are located in the region of the external occipital protuberance. These points are usually needled for amplifying the therapeutic responses to acupuncture and can be needled in every treatment session.

The tinnitus master key point is located in the area of the Du-16 acupuncture point (below the occipital protuberances and above the C1 vertebra). This point is needled when treating patients with tinnitus using the four-point needling combination for treating tinnitus (see Chapter 3). It can also be effective in treating patients suffering from vertigo and dizziness, or nausea.

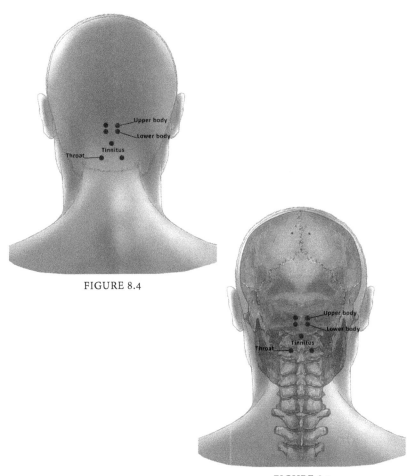

FIGURE 8.4

FIGURE 8.5

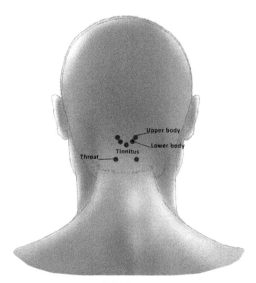

FIGURE 8.6

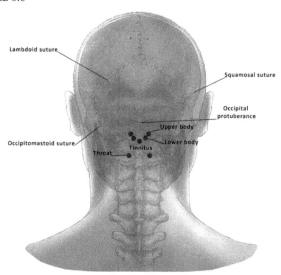

FIGURE 8.7

Two bilateral points, a master key point of the upper body and a master key point of the lower body, are located in cavities or notches that are approximately 0.5 cm lateral to the external occipital protuberance. Needling the point that is located in the upper part of the notch can amplify the therapeutic responses to acupuncture of the upper body. Needling the point that is located in the lower part of the notch can amplify the therapeutic responses to acupuncture of the lower part of the body.

- **Master key point of the upper body** (above the diaphragm): This point is located in the upper part of the cavity (notch), and needling this point amplifies the therapeutic responses to acupuncture of the upper part of the body.

- **Master key point of the lower body** (below the diaphragm): This point is located in the upper part of the cavity (notch), and needling this point will amplify the therapeutic responses to acupuncture of the lower part of the body.

In many cases, I concomitantly needle these two points to treat disorders of the lower extremities, such as foot drop, neuropathic pain of the legs, paralyses, and heel spurs. Needling these two master key points will exert an effect on the patient's balance and vision.

- **Master key point of the throat**: This point is located beneath the transverse process of the C1 vertebra (Huatuo Jiaji acupuncture points between the C1 and C2 vertebrae). Needling this point can be used to amplify the therapeutic responses to acupuncture when treating hoarseness, laryngitis, thyroid disorders, parathyroid disorders, and swallowing.

Additional points

Over the years, additional needling points were added to the existing YNSA points. Each of these added points has no diagnostic zone or is associated with a specific category of YNSA points.

Oral points and diagnostic zone

The oral points are two bilateral points that are located on the edge of the eye socket in an area between the middle part of the eyebrow (UB-2 acupuncture point) and the nasofrontal suture (nasal bridge). These points are needled for all oral problems, and their diagnostic zone is located over the sternoclavicular joint (SCJ).

Note: According to the nasal acupuncture microsystem, the oral points can also be used to treat shoulder pain and shoulder disorders.

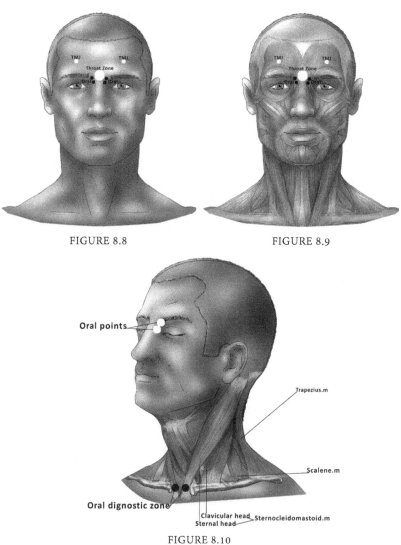

FIGURE 8.8   FIGURE 8.9

FIGURE 8.10

Throat area

The throat area is located between the Yin Tang acupuncture point, the nasofrontal suture (nasal bridge), and the two eyebrows (UB-2 acupuncture point). The indications for needling this area are conditions of the throat and vocal cords and swallowing problems.

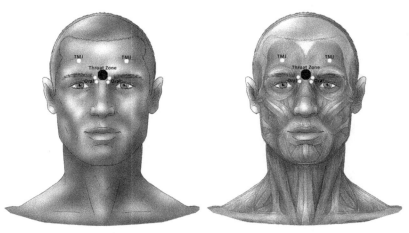

FIGURE 8.11   FIGURE 8.12

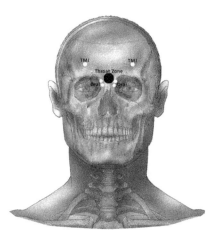

FIGURE 8.13

Foot point

The foot point is located on the zygomatic arch on the front edge of the sideburn. The indications for needling this point are foot problems, such as ankle sprain, paralysis, foot drop, or plantar fasciitis.

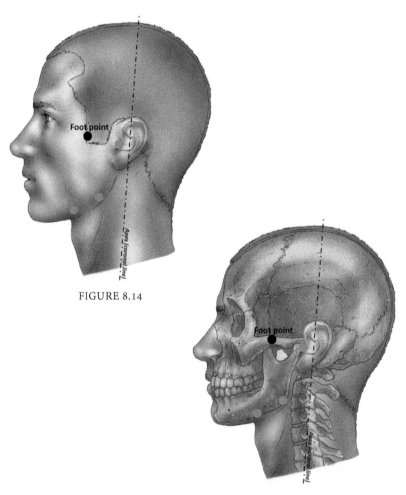

FIGURE 8.14

FIGURE 8.15

Extra knee point

The extra knee point is located on the hairline midway between the basic B point and basic C point. The indication for needling this point is acute knee pain.

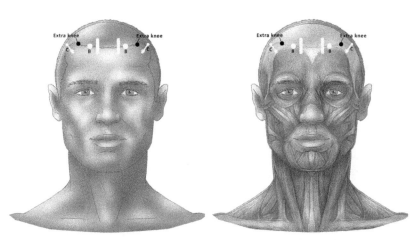

FIGURE 8.16   FIGURE 8.17

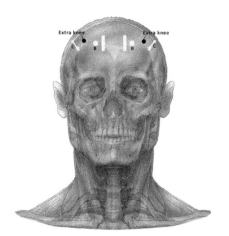

FIGURE 8.18

Extra lumbar point

The extra lumbar point is located on the mandible, half way between the angle of the mandible and the center of the chin. The indication for needling this point is lower back pain.

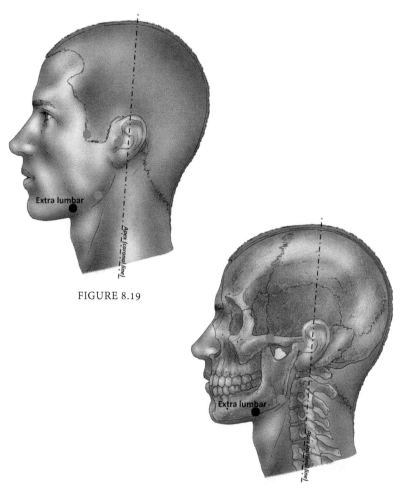

FIGURE 8.19

FIGURE 8.20

Extra shoulder point

The extra shoulder point is located on the mandible bone between the mandibular angle and the mastoid muscles. The indications for needling this point are an inability to internally rotate or horizontally extend the shoulder.

Note: In some cases, the practitioner can needle this point to treat acute knee pain.

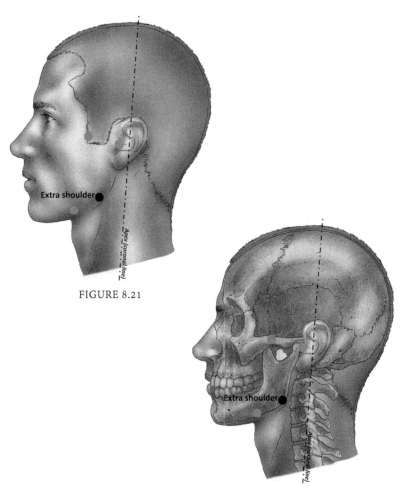

FIGURE 8.21

FIGURE 8.22

Gastrocnemius muscle point

This point is located in a notch on the posterior side of the TMJ and overlaps the cervical spine region of the I somatotope. The indication for needling this point is spasm of the gastrocnemius muscle. Needling this point can be used to treat heel spurs and plantar fasciitis.

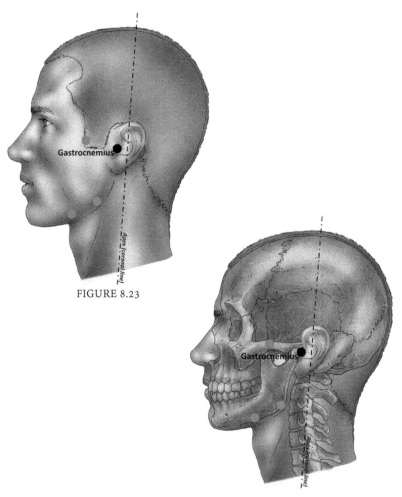

FIGURE 8.23

FIGURE 8.24

Soleus muscle area

The Achilles tendon is the conjoined tendon of the gastrocnemius and soleus muscles. The medial and lateral soleus muscle areas are located where the soleus muscle becomes the Achilles tendon, approximately 3–4 cm above the malleus bone. One point is located on the medial side of the shin (around the KID-7 acupuncture point), and the second point is located on the lateral side of the shin (around the UB-59 acupuncture point). The patient should be examined for sensitivity of the KID-7 acupuncture point (medial) and UB-59 acupuncture point (lateral) prior to needling. The indications for needling the medial area are problems with flexing the palms of the hands. The indications for needling the lateral area are problems with extending the palms of the hands.

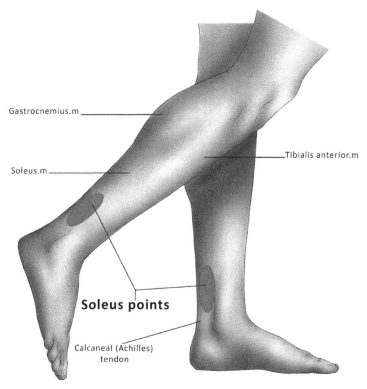

FIGURE 8.25

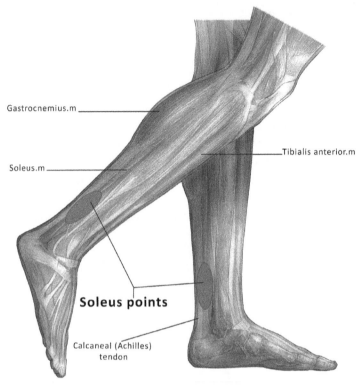

FIGURE 8.26

ZS point and diagnostic zone

Note: Between 2005 and 2007, Dr Dorothea Zeise-Suess discovered a new needling point (ZS) for treating disturbances of the female hormonal system. This point was subsequently validated by Dr Yamamoto and has been added to the YNSA points.

The ZS needling point is located over the anterior temporal bone, approximately 1 cm below the mid-forehead line and approximately 1–2 cm posterior to the hairline. The diagnostic zone for the ZS needling point can be located by palpating an area that is located between the posterior end of the clavicular division of the sternocleidomastoid muscle (SCM) (Kidney neck diagnostic zone) and the ST-12 acupuncture point, which is located in the supraclavicular fossa, and approximately 5 cm lateral to the sternoclavicular joint (SCJ).

The indications for needling the ZS point are disturbances of the female hormonal system and infertility, amenorrhea, dysmenorrhea, hot flashes, hypermenorrhea, menometrorrhagia, and climacteric syndrome.

Palpation and comments: Pressure is applied towards the scapula using the thumb.

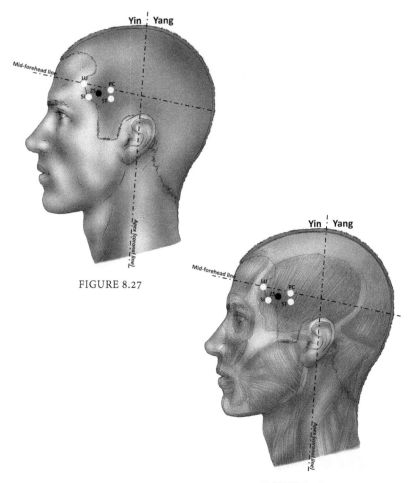

FIGURE 8.27

FIGURE 8.28

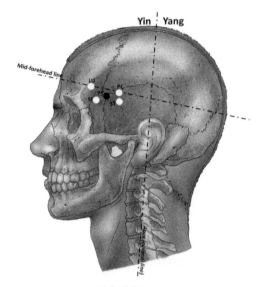

FIGURE 8.29

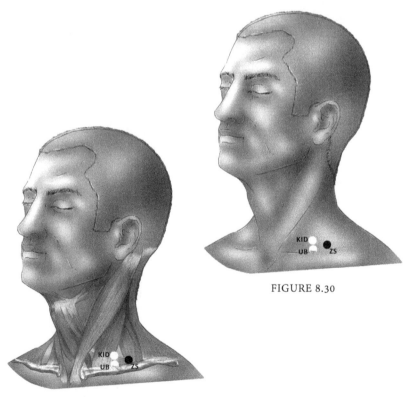

FIGURE 8.30

FIGURE 8.31

Speech pathology points: Broca and Wernicke's needling points

Broca's area and Wernicke's area are two anatomical areas that underlie speech and are located in the left cerebral cortex of the brain. Broca's aphasia is a type of aphasia characterized by partial loss of the ability to produce language (spoken, motor speech, or written communication known as written speech), although comprehension generally remains intact. Wernicke's aphasia, which is also known as receptive aphasia, sensory aphasia, or posterior aphasia, is a type of aphasia in which individuals have difficulty understanding written and spoken language.

The **Broca** needling point is located in the anterior temporal region between the PI and ST Ypsilon points on the Yin aspect of the scalp. The indication for needling the Broca point is treatment of motor speech disorders.

The **Wernicke** needling point is located in the posterior temporal region between the PI and ST Ypsilon points on the Yang aspect of the scalp. The indication for needling Wernicke's point is to treat language processing or comprehension disorders.

Note: When treating aphasia, I recommend needling the Broca and Wernicke points bilaterally as well as needling the mouth sensory point, throat point, and cranial nerve 11 point.

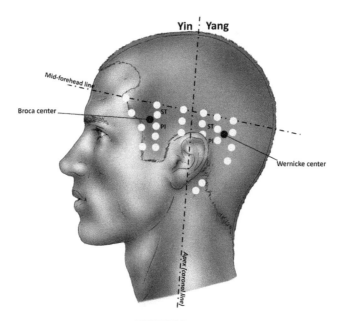

FIGURE 8.32

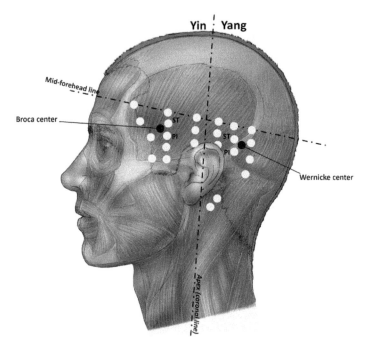

FIGURE 8.33

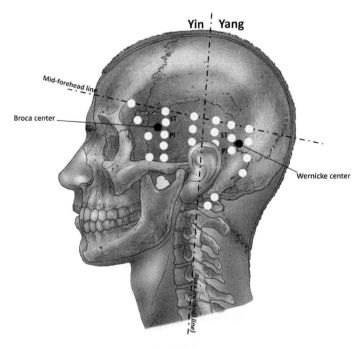

FIGURE 8.34

J and K somatotopes

The J and K somatotopes were developed as needling points in YNSA at the same time as the basic points were developed. These two somatotopes extend along the sagittal suture. The J somatotope is located on the sagittal suture on the Yin aspect, and the K somatotope is located on the Yang aspect of the sagittal suture.

The J somatotope extends from the vertex of the skull (upper surface of the head) (head region of the somatotope) to the anterior hairline (foot region of the somatotope). The K somatotope extends from the vertex of the skull (head region of the somatotope) and continues posterior to the lambdoid suture (foot region of the somatotope).

The differences between the J and K somatotopes are:

- *Needling the J somatotope* will treat the anterior aspect of the body.

- *Needling the K somatotope* will treat the posterior body.

In practice, needling the J and K somatotopes will be used to treat the foot region.

- Needling the J somatotope is more effective than needling the K somatotope when treating conditions of the dorsal surface (upper surface) of the foot, such as drop foot, ankle sprains, Morton's neuroma (intermetatarsal neuroma), and shin splint.

- Needling the K somatotope is more effective than needling the J somatotope when treating conditions of the plantar surface (bottom surface) of the foot such as heel spurs, plantar fasciitis, and other conditions of the foot's plantar surface, and burning sensation of the heel.

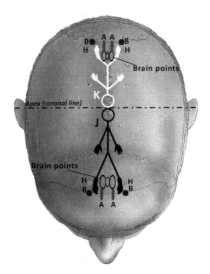

FIGURE 8.35

Vertebral somatotope

Needling the vertebral somatotope is mainly done for treating musculoskeletal trauma and musculoskeletal pain. The vertebral somatotope is located on the transverse process of the vertebrae between vertebrae C6 to T2.

Each vertebra will treat a different region on the spine when needled (lumbar, thoracic, or cervical):

- Needling the space between C6 and C7 is done for treating disorders of the lumbar spine.

- Needling the space between C7 and T1 is done for treating disorders of the thoracic spine.

- Needling the space between T1 and T2 is done for treating disorders of the cervical spine.

Note: When locating sensitivity in these areas, you will need to apply approximately 1 kg (2.2 lbs) of pressure and palpate as close as possible to the center of the spinal vertebra.

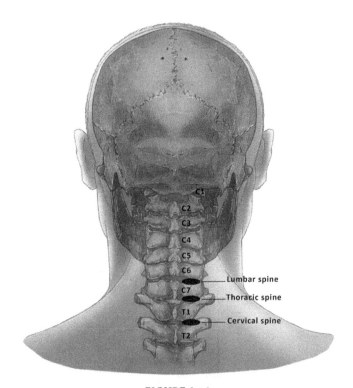

FIGURE 8.36

Chest somatotope

Needling the chest somatotope is mainly done when treating musculoskeletal injuries. This somatotope is located on the lateral borders of the sternum down to the 7th rib.

The side that will be needled in this somatotope is ipsilateral to the patient's complaint.

The location of the head region in the chest somatotope is on the jugular notch.

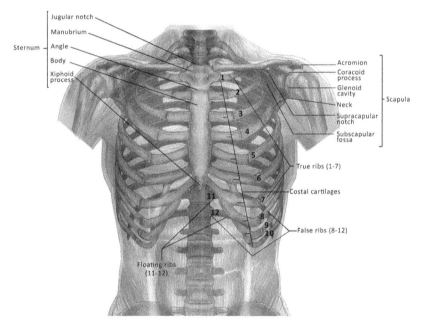

FIGURE 8.37

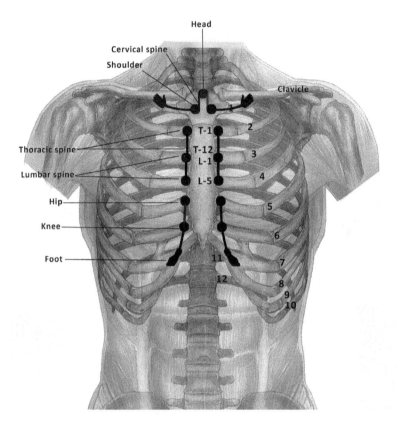

FIGURE 8.38

The cervical spine region of the chest somatotope is a 2 cm vertical line that starts around the sternal notch area (representation of the C1 vertebra) and continues approximately 2 cm below the sternal notch area (representation of the C7 vertebra). This 2 cm line is located in the center of the sternum and is needled to treat disorders of the cervical spine.

- The location of the **upper extremity** in the chest somatotope is between the costal cartilage of the first rib (representation of the shoulder region) and the point where the first rib and the clavicular bone (representation of the palm of the hand) meet. This line is needled to treat disorders of the upper extremities.

- The location of the **thoracic spine** region in the chest somatotope is on the lateral borders of the sternum between the costal cartilage of the second rib (representation of the T1 vertebra) and the costal cartilage of the third rib (representation of the T12 vertebra). This line is needled to treat disorders of the thoracic spine.

- The location of the **lumbar spine** region in the chest somatotope is on the lateral borders of the sternum between the costal cartilage of the fourth rib (representation of the L1 vertebra) and the costal cartilage of the fifth rib (representation of the L5 vertebra). This line is needled to treat disorders of the lumbar spine.

- The location of the **sacral, hip, and coccyx** region of the chest somatotope is on the costal cartilage of the sixth rib. This line is needled to treat disorders of the sacrum, hip, and coccyx.

- The location of the **knee-foot** region of the chest somatotope is between the costal cartilage of the seventh rib (knee region) and the integration (costal margin of seventh and eighth rib) point of the seventh rib (representation of the foot region) with the eighth rib. This area is needled when the patient has trauma to the knee, hip, or foot.

Note: When needling this somatotope, be very cautious in order to not penetrate the lungs.

Case Studies

* * * * * *

The objective of this chapter is to improve the clinical utility of YNSA for practitioners. To this end, this chapter presents three groups of case studies. The first group comprises examples of using YNSA to treat the symptoms, especially pain, of different disorders. The second group comprises examples in which elbow diagnosis is done before applying YNSA. The third group comprises examples in which neck, abdomen, and elbow diagnosis is done when needling the Ypsilon, cranial nerve, and basic points.

Group 1 using YNSA to treat symptoms
Case 1
A 35-year-old man with severe back pain in his lower left side and spasm of the gastrocnemius muscle on the right side.

Case history
A healthy 35-year-old man with no history of illness woke up one morning with severe lower back pain on his left side and a spasm of the gastrocnemius muscle in his right leg. He thought he had made a mistake by sleeping with the air conditioner on because it was very hot and humid, and he had not covered himself when sleeping. When he arose, he decided to go for a run because he thought running would relieve the back pain and muscle spasm. When he started running, the pain became more intense and he began limping. He then stopped running and did some stretching in the hope that it would relieve the back pain and reduce the tension in his back and gastrocnemius muscle.

Treatment

The points that were palpated and then needled were (i) the F point, (ii) the I somatotope where the gastrocnemius muscle needling point is located, and (iii) the extra D point on the ipsilateral (same) side of the symptoms. These three points were palpated and then needled for treating disorders of the musculoskeletal system of the lumbar spine and lower extremities.

Palpation of the D point, the extra D point, and the F point on the right side revealed increased sensitivity of the F point. After applying pressure on the F point, the patient was asked to bend forward to determine whether the back pain was relieved before needling the point. After bending forward, the patient reported improvement in his forward bend and pain relief in the lower back. After needling the F point, the patient reported, "My lower back pain is better [has lessened], but I still feel a slight pain in my lower back." A second palpation of the extra D point revealed sensitivity of the point. After applying pressure to the point, the patient reported relief of the back pain and reduced tension of the back muscles. Accordingly, the extra D point on the right side was needled. Since there was still pain and tension in the patient's gastrocnemius muscle, the I somatotope where the reflection of the gastrocnemius muscle is represented in the I somatotope. This palpation revealed another sensitive point in the area of the gastrocnemius muscle of the I somatotope. When this point was needled, the patient reported relief of the pain and tension in his gastrocnemius muscle. The patient was then asked to do a quick 1-minute run with the needles in place to see whether he still had any symptoms of back pain and muscle pain. After the run, the patient reported that he was pain-free. The needles were then withdrawn and the patient subsequently reported that he was able to run without any pain.

Case 2

A 45-year-old woman with severe menstrual cramps in her lower abdomen just before and during her menstruation.

Case history

A 45-year-old woman complained of severe menstrual cramps in her lower abdomen that disappeared after three days of menstruation. She reported that these symptoms had begun during the last year and recurred at each menstruation. She also complained that she frequently had fever and flu symptoms, pain and weakness of the lower and upper extremities, and a cold feeling in her hands and feet. She also complained of headaches around the occipital region of the head when the weather was cold.

Treatment

The treatment comprised a combination of YNSA and traditional Chinese acupuncture. The patient initially presented on the first day of a three-day episode of menstrual cramps. She complained of abdominal pain on the left and right side and a severe headache in the occipital region on the right side of her head. In order to feel more comfortable, relieve her headache, and allow her to relax, the basic A and B points on the right side were needled to treat her headache and the pain in her neck and upper back. After 2–3 minutes, she reported that she felt the headache pain had subsided greatly and felt more relaxed. Since she also reported that the pain of her menstrual cramps had subsided but not disappeared, the basic D point was then needled bilaterally in order to treat lower abdominal pain. After 2 minutes, she reported considerable pain relief in her lower abdomen.

Since the patient reported incomplete relief of her symptoms, she was then examined using traditional Chinese medicine. She was diagnosed as having a disorder of the Tai Yang channel that could be treated by needling the KID-2 and HT-8 acupuncture points in the Shao Ying channel because needling these points would relieve all her symptoms. About 15 minutes after treating the Tai Yang channel, she reported that the headache and pain of her menstrual cramps were gone. She returned for five 45-minute treatments that comprised tonifying the Tai Yang channel and needling the basic A, B, and D points. At each presentation, she reported progressive alleviation of her symptoms that disappeared after the fifth treatment.

Case 3

A 10-week pregnant 32-year-old woman with loss of appetite, nausea, heartburn, and vomiting.

Case history

A 10-week pregnant 32-year-old woman complained of losing weight and feeling weak because she had no appetite and the thought of food caused her to vomit. The symptoms started after the third week of her pregnancy.

Treatment

The treatment comprised bilateral needling of the basic D, E, and throat points. The D point was needled bilaterally to (i) treat the lower abdominal pain, and (ii) reduce (slow) the stomach's motility and prevent excessive production of stomach acid, which could be causing the nausea, heart burn, and bilious attacks. The E point was needled bilaterally to prevent the reflux of stomach acidity into the esophagus, thereby treating the heartburn. The throat point was needled to treat the feeling of nausea, the need to vomit, and biliousness.

Approximately 10 minutes after needling these points, the woman reported alleviation of her symptoms. The needles that were inserted to stimulate the D and E points were withdrawn and replaced with intradermal needles before sending her home. The needle that was inserted to stimulate the throat point was withdrawn and not replaced with an intradermal needle. After three days, the woman reported that she was feeling better, was eating again, and no longer had the feeling of needing to vomit. The intradermal needles were removed after one week.

Group 2 using elbow diagnosis in YNSA
Case 1
A 50-year-old man with a spinal cord injury at the level of cervical vertebra 5 due to a diving accident.

Case history
The patient was a 50-year-old man who had been hospitalized because of decompression sickness that developed when he was scuba diving. He was comatose when he was placed in the decompression chamber. When he regained consciousness five days later, he could not move his lower extremities and was diagnosed with a spinal cord injury at the level of cervical vertebra 5. Two days after regaining consciousness, he was able to move his legs, and ten days later he was able to move his legs when sitting. On examination, there was spasticity in the hip region and quadricep muscles, which left him leaning forward and unable to walk. Nonetheless, he could raise his feet when he sat down.

Treatment
The treatment comprised needling the basic A point because the patient was unable to walk due to damage to the cervical spine and spasticity in

his hips and quadriceps. The basic B point was also needled to block the firing of those neurons (nerve cells) that were causing the leg muscles to contract and the spasticity in his legs.

Examination of the palms of the hands revealed a purple color of the right palm that indicates disruption of the flow of qi and blood on the right side. Palpation of the elbow diagnostic zone revealed increased sensitivity of the cervical spine region on the left side. Accordingly, the A point on the left side of the scalp was needled because needling this point is done to treat neck pain and nerve damage in the cervical spine, and to improve the movement of the cervical spine. A repeat palpation of the cervical spine diagnostic zone in the left elbow revealed reduced sensitivity, which was also reported by the patient.

Since the diagnostic zone of the cervical spine on the left elbow was still sensitive, the basic B point was then needled. After this needling, a repeat palpation of the cervical spine diagnostic zone in the left elbow revealed no sensitivity. The patient was able to stand upright and walk with a walking assistance device. After needling the basic A and B points on the left side, a repeat bilateral palpation of the LI-4 (He Gu) acupuncture point revealed no sensitivity on the left and right sides. The absence of sensitivity of the LI-4 acupuncture point indicates that the disorder has been treated and there is no need to needle other points. After 30 minutes, examination of the palms of his hands revealed that the purple color of the right side had disappeared: the color of the two palms was becoming red and vivid. The needles that were inserted at the A and B points were then withdrawn so as not to overstimulate the patient.

The acupuncture treatment, which comprised twice-weekly needling of the basic A and B points for 60 minutes, continued for three months. During this period, the patient improved: he was able to stand upright and walk about 100 meters before needing to rest.

Case 2

A 33-year-old woman with an episodic exacerbation of multiple sclerosis (MS) symptoms (an acute MS attack).

Case history

The patient was a 33-year-old woman with MS, which was diagnosed two years earlier when she complained of feeling weak and unstable while standing. Although she was under medical care, she had an acute MS attack. After the attack, she displayed hemiataxia on the right side with a feeling of weakness in her right leg. Her hands and arms shook when raised and she was unable to touch her nose.

Treatment

Examination of the palms of the patient's hands revealed that the left palm was paler than the right palm. Palpation of the LI-4 (He Gu) acupuncture point and the cerebellum diagnostic zone revealed increased sensitivity on the right side. The cerebellum zone on the Yang aspect of the scalp was needled because needling points on the Yang aspect is more effective than needling points on the Yin aspect in MS patients. After needling the cerebellum diagnostic zone, a repeat palpation of the cerebellum diagnostic zone in the right elbow revealed that the sensitivity had subsided. This lessening of sensitivity indicates that the correct point had been needled.

Palpation of the basal ganglion diagnostic zone on the left side revealed increased sensitivity. Accordingly, the basal ganglia needling point on the left side on the Yang aspect of the scalp was needled. After needling this point, a repeat palpation of the ganglion diagnostic zone in the left elbow revealed that the sensitivity had subsided. This lessening of sensitivity indicates that the correct point had been needled.

Palpation of the lumbar diagnostic zone on the left side revealed increased sensitivity. Accordingly, the region of the lumbar spine and the foot of somatotope I on the left side was needled. Repeat palpation of the lumbar diagnostic zone on the left side revealed that the sensitivity had subsided. This lessening of sensitivity indicates that the correct point had been needled.

A repeat palpation of the LI-4 acupuncture point on the left and right sides revealed no sensitivity, which indicates that the treatment was successful and there was no need to needle additional points.

When the patient stood up, she reported that standing was no longer difficult and she had more control of her legs. Moreover, she was able to take a few steps with the help of a physiotherapist. Nevertheless, she reported that she felt that her right knee kept folding and collapsing. Accordingly, the basic H point on the right side was needled. After needling this point, the patient reported that control of her right knee and right foot had improved, she could control her walking, and there was less shaking in her hands and arms.

The patient received one-hour acupuncture treatments of YNSA twice weekly for two months, in addition to receiving twice-weekly physiotherapy. Over this period, she improved: she was able to stand and walk with a mild degree of ataxia, but her hands still shook when trying to touch her nose. She reported that she had not experienced any acute MS attacks in the 12 months after completing treatment.

Group 3 using elbow, neck, and abdominal diagnosis in YNSA
Case 1
A 42-year-old woman with diabetes, weakness of the right leg, difficulty in urinating, and chronic pain in her lower back and neck.

Case history
The patient was a 42-year-old woman with high blood pressure, diabetes, and sleep apnea. She had undergone back surgery for a prolapsed disc between lumbar vertebrae 4 and 5. The surgery was not completely successful because she was left with weakness of the right foot and difficulty in urinating. She also complained of chronic pain in her lower back and neck.

Treatment
The treatment comprised needling (i) the LIV point because palpation of the liver diagnostic zone in the neck revealed sensitivity that occurs when the patient has a sleep disorder (needling the LIV point improves the patient's sleep and activates the parasympathetic nervous system), (ii) the PI Ypsilon point because palpation of the spleen diagnostic zone in the neck revealed sensitivity, which occurs in diabetic patients (needling this point improves pancreatic function and lowers blood sugar [glucose] levels), and (iii) the KID Ypsilon point because palpation of the kidney diagnostic zone in the neck revealed sensitivity.

Examination of the palms of the patient's hands revealed a purple color of the left palm. Palpation of the LI-4 (He Gu) acupuncture point on the right side revealed increased sensitivity. Palpation of the kidney zone of the neck diagnostic zone revealed that the left kidney zone was more sensitive than the right kidney zone (the kidney diagnostic zone was palpated to determine which side of the neck will be used for diagnosing and needling). After needling the KID point, the kidney diagnostic zone was palpated again and revealed that its sensitivity had lessened.

Palpation of the neck diagnostic zone also revealed sensitivity in the liver, spleen, and urinary bladder zones. Accordingly, the LIV, PI, and UB Ypsilon points on the left side were needled. After needling these points, a repeat palpation of the liver, spleen, and urinary bladder zones in the neck diagnostic zone revealed no sensitivity of the three zones, which indicates that the treatment, namely needling the LIV, PI, and UB Ypsilon acupuncture points, was successful and there was no need to needle additional points.

After needling the LIV and PI Ypsilon points on the left side, a repeat palpation of the LI-4 acupuncture point revealed that the point was still sensitive. Palpation of the left cervical spine diagnostic zone in the elbow was sensitive.

Palpation of the basic A point and the region of the cervical spine of the I somatotope on the left side revealed that the A point was more sensitive than the region of the cervical spine in the I somatotope. Accordingly, the basic A point was needled. Since a repeat bilateral palpation of the LI-4 acupuncture point revealed no sensitivity, it was not necessary to needle more points.

After 40 minutes, a repeat examination of the palms of the patient's hands revealed that the color of both palms was even. Therefore, the needles were withdrawn (when the color of the palms of the hands is the same, it is an indication that the needles can be withdrawn). When the patient now walked, her gait had visibly improved and she reported that the weakness in her foot had lessened. The next day, she reported that there was less weakness in her legs and she had had a good night's sleep.

After the first treatment, the patient reported no difficulty in urinating. She then received ten twice-weekly 45-minute treatments of YNSA. After the tenth treatment, she reported that the weakness in her legs had disappeared and she was sleeping well at night ("I put my head on the pillow and close my eyes and I am out for the night. When I open my eyes it is morning, and I feel refreshed and ready for a new day").

Although she thinks that her sleep apnea has been resolved, at the time of writing she arranged to be re-examined in a sleep laboratory to determine whether it has actually been resolved. She changed her diet to a ketogenic diet (high-fat, adequate-protein, low-carbohydrate diet) after a dietitian instructed her to change her diet in order to treat her diabetes and control her blood pressure.

About three months after the treatments, she reported that her blood sugar levels and blood pressure were normal: her doctor has lowered the dose of her diabetic medications and withdrawn treatment for blood pressure control.

Case 2

A 75-year-old man who was referred by an orthopedic surgeon for treatment of a partial tear of the supraspinous tendon in the right shoulder.

Case history

The patient was a 75-year-old man who complained that a partial tear of the supraspinous tendon which was causing severe pain in his right shoulder and difficulty in raising his right arm. He also complained that the pain increased when he was sleeping and interrupted his sleep.

Treatment

The treatment comprised needling (i) the PC Ypsilon point because needling this point exerts an effect on the supraspinous muscle and tendon, (ii) the GB Ypsilon point because needling this point exerts an effect on the scapular spine, thereby enabling improved rotation of the shoulder, (iii) the UB Ypsilon point because needling this point causes relaxation of the muscles in the upper back and neck, thereby releasing tension in the rotator cuff muscles and allowing the shoulder to move freely, (iv) the SI Ypsilon point because the small intestine diagnostic zone in the neck was sensitive, and (v) the SI channel was needled because this channel passes through the scapular spine and a disorder of this channel causes shoulder pain and affects movement of the scapula.

On presentation, the patient was able to raise his right arm to the level of the right shoulder. Examination of the palms of his hands revealed a purple color of the right palm.

Palpation of the LI-4 (He Gu) acupuncture point revealed that the left side was more sensitive than the right side (when the patient's complaint is above the diaphragm, palpation of the LI-4 acupuncture point will determine the side of the neck to palpate for diagnosing and needling of the Ypsilon or cranial nerve points).

Palpation of the left side of the neck diagnostic zone revealed sensitivity of the pericardium and urinary bladder zones. Accordingly, the PC and UB Ypsilon points were needled.

A repeat palpation of the pericardium and urinary bladder zones on the left side of the neck revealed that the sensitivity had lessened and indicates that the correct points were needled. When he was asked to raise his arm, the patient could raise it above the height of the shoulder.

A repeat palpation of the LI-4 acupuncture point revealed that the right side was more sensitive than the left side.

A repeat palpation of the neck diagnostic zone on the right side revealed that the gallbladder and small intestine diagnostic zones were sensitive. Accordingly, the GB and SI Ypsilon points on the right side were needled.

After needling the GB and SI Ypsilon points, a repeat palpation of the gallbladder and small intestine diagnostic zones on the right side in the neck revealed that the sensitivity had lessened and indicates that the correct points were needled.

When he was then asked to raise his arm, the patient was able to raise it above his head and felt no pain.

A repeat bilateral palpation of the LI-4 acupuncture point revealed no sensitivity on the left and right sides. This lack of sensitivity indicates that the disorder had been treated correctly and there was no need for additional needling.

After 30 minutes, an examination of the palms revealed the same color of his left and right palms. Accordingly, the needles were withdrawn from the scalp. After this single treatment, the patient reported that he had no more shoulder pain and his sleep was pain-free.

Appendix

• • • • • •

Basic points

Point	Location	Indications
A	Approximately 1 cm lateral to the sagittal line of the face A 2 cm vertical line that runs from 1 cm above the hairline to 1 cm below the hairline	Neck problems (cervical vertebrae C1–C7); cranial problems (dental pain, eyes, ears, swallowing, and throat)
B	Approximately 2 cm lateral to the sagittal line The point is on the natural hairline	Problems of the neck, upper shoulder, and shoulder blade (upper trapezius muscle), problems of and pain in the nape, sore throat, problems of the thyroid gland
C	The line begins 1 cm above the hairline and continues 1 cm below the hairline at an approximate angle of 45° to the nasal bridge. The mid-point of this 2 cm line is the GB-13 acupuncture point (on the superior border of the temporalis muscle)	For any neurological problems between the shoulder and hand
D	An imaginary line that runs from the outer corner of the eye to the ear base and crosses the front edge of the sideburn (approximately 1 cm superior to the zygomatic bone) The extra D point is just below the ear base where the face meets the ear	All problems of the diaphragm and below; orthopedic and neurological problems of the pelvis, legs, and lower back; gynecological problems; bowel and bladder problems

Point	Location	Indications
E	An oblique 2 cm line that starts 1 cm lateral to the midline above the eyebrow	Problems of the thoracic vertebrae; cardiovascular problems; breathing difficulties and respiratory conditions; conditions of the liver, stomach, and diaphragm
F	The point is located on the striking out point of the mastoid bone (approx 1.5 cm above the mastoid process)	All types of sciatica; problems of the piriformis muscle
G	In the arch about 3 mm above the basic D point on the Yin aspect at the edge of the mastoid bone on the Yang aspect	Knee problems due to direct trauma of the knee; acute knee problems in the Yin aspect; chronic knee problems in the Yang aspect
H	Approximately 1 cm above the basic B point	Lower back problems; very effective for knee problems

Sensory organ points

Organ	Location	Indications
Eye	About 1 cm below the line of the basic A point	All ophthalmic disturbances and pain, inflammation, itching, redness, loss of vision, glaucoma, cataract, lazy eye, dryness of the eye, and loss of function of the muscles that surround the eye
Nose	About 2 cm below the line of the basic A point in the middle of the forehead	Loss of smell, nasal polyps, sinusitis, rhinitis, nasal congestion, runny nose, and allergies
Mouth	About 1 cm above the midpoint of the line of the basic E point	Speech problems, motor aphasia, toothache, inflammation, and infections of the oral cavity, oral ulcers, and oral sores
Ear	Continuation of the line of the basic C point towards the nasal bridge of the nose between the eye and nose points	Tinnitus, fluid buildup in the ear (otitis media), inflammation and infections of the ear, sudden deafness, auricular pain, and loss of balance

Throat zone	This area is located between the Yin Tang point, the nasal bridge, and UB-2 acupuncture point	The indications for needling this area are conditions of the throat and vocal cords and for swallowing difficulties
Oral points	These are two bilateral points that are located on the edge of the eye socket in an area between UB-2 acupuncture point and the nasal bridge	These points are needled for all oral problems, and their diagnostic zone is located over the sternoclavicular joint
TMJ	This is a bilateral point that is located on the pupil line approximately 1 cm above the eyebrow	TMJ disorders

Neck diagnostic zones

Organ and channel	Location	Comments
Kidney (KID)	Posterior division of the sternocleidomastoid muscle (SCM) and clavicle	Pressure is applied towards the scapula using the thumb
Urinary Bladder (UB)	Same location as the Kidney diagnostic zone and partly behind the clavicle	The thumb is pressed down and posterior to the clavicle
Liver (LIV)	The center of the SCM at the level of the throat midway between the clavicle and mandibular angle	The thumb is moved back and forth across the SCM with a very gentle touch
Pericardium (PC)	The anterior division of the SCM at the level of the Liver diagnostic zone; the point is located on the anterior borders of the SCM	The thumb is moved in an anterior direction Pressure needs to be applied on the anterior border of the SCM
Heart (HT)	The anterior border of the SCM at about a 45° angle above the Liver diagnostic zone; the point is located on the anterior border of the SCM	The thumb is moved at a 45° angle in an upward direction. Pressure needs to be applied on the anterior border of the SCM

Organ and channel	Location	Comments
Gallbladder (GB)	The anterior border of the SCM at about a 45° angle below the Liver diagnostic zone	Move the thumb downwards in a 45° angle direction Pressure needs to be applied on the anterior border of the SCM
Small Intestine (SI)	The meeting point of the mandibular angle and the anterior border of the trapezius muscle (in the area of the SJ-16 acupuncture point)	Gentle pressure is needed when palpating
Stomach (ST)	On the vertical fibers of the trapezius muscle midway between the Large Intestine neck diagnostic zone and the Small Intestine neck diagnostic zone (This point is located at the same level as the Liver neck diagnostic zone on the trapezius muscle)	Gentle pressure is needed when palpating
Spleen/ Pancreas (PI)	Anterior to the vertical fibers of the trapezius muscle midway between the Large Intestine neck diagnostic zone and the Small Intestine neck diagnostic zone (This point is located at the same level as the Large Intestine neck diagnostic zone on the trapezius muscle)	The thumb is moved from the Stomach diagnostic zone The pressure can change from gentle to strong
Large Intestine (LI)	On the trapezius muscle where the horizontal fibers and vertical fibers of the trapezius muscle merge (where the neck and shoulder meet) Located slightly medial and slightly anterior to the GB-21 acupuncture point	The thumb should roll on the muscle Gentle pressure is needed

San Jiao (SJ)	The anterior border of the trapezius muscle where the horizontal and vertical fibers of the trapezius muscle meet	The thumb is moved from the Large Intestine diagnostic test zone anterior to the trapezius muscle
Lung (LU)	Lateral to thyroid cartilage	Apply gentle pressure to both sides of the thyroid
ZS	Approximately 1 cm lateral to the Kidney diagnostic zone	Pressure is applied towards the scapula using the thumb
Oral	Over the sternoclavicular joint (SCJ)	Press the thumb into the joint

Abdomen diagnostic zones

Organ and channel	Location	Comments
Kidney (KID)	Bilaterally above the pelvic bone in the area of the GB-27 acupuncture point (the Kidney diagnostic zone is the only diagnostic zone that is located bilaterally)	Around GB-27 acupuncture point
Urinary Bladder (UB)	2–3 cm above the center of the pubic symphysis	Around Ren-3, 4 acupuncture points
Pericardium (PC)	1–2 cm below the heart zone	Around Ren-14 acupuncture point
Heart (HT)	1–2 cm below the xiphoid process	Around Ren-15 acupuncture point
Stomach (ST)	6–7 cm above the umbilicus	Around Ren-12 acupuncture point
San Jiao (SJ)	2–3 cm below the umbilicus	Around Ren-7 acupuncture point
Small Intestine (SI)	Approximately 6 cm from the right side of the umbilicus on a 45° downward line	Around ST-28 acupuncture point
Spleen/ Pancreas (PI)	Directly below the left costal margin	Around SP-16 acupuncture point, on the left side

Organ and channel	Location	Comments
Lung (LU)	45° upward line from the umbilicus between the right costal margin and the umbilicus	Around ST-22 acupuncture point on the left side
Liver (LIV)	45° upward line from the umbilicus between the left costal margin and the umbilicus	Around ST-22 acupuncture point on the right side
Gallbladder (GB)	Directly below the right costal margin	Around SP-16 acupuncture point, on the right side
Large Intestine (LI)	45° downward line from the umbilicus, approximately 6 cm from the left side of the umbilicus	Around ST-28 acupuncture point

Brain zones

Zone	Location	Indications
Cerebral	A 2 cm vertical line that begins 1 cm above the hairline and about 1 cm lateral to the midline	All acute and chronic neurological problems, short- and long-term motor problems, psychiatric disorders, attention deficit disorder, attention deficit hyperactivity disorder, sleep and memory disorders, and hormonal disorders
Cerebellum	A 1 cm vertical line that begins about 3 cm above the hairline and overlies the lower part of the cerebral diagnostic zone	Problems of balance, spatial orientation, coordination learning, and timing

| Basal ganglia | This zone has two locations, old and new:

1. Old location: approximately 3 cm vertical line that runs from about 1 cm to 4 cm into the hairline, located on the mid-sagittal line (sagittal suture)

2. New location based on elbow diagnosis: approximately 3 cm vertical line that runs from about 1 cm to 4 cm into the hairline, located approximately 0.5 cm lateral to the mid-sagittal line (midway between the A point and the mid-sagittal line) | Loss of control of voluntary motor movements, and movement disorders (hyperkinetic disorders) |

Cranial nerve points

Cranial nerve number	Chinese medicine organ and channel association to the cranial nerve	Latin name	Western medicine function
1	Kidney (KID)	Olfactorius	The sensory nerve of smell
2	Urinary Bladder (UB)	Opticus	The nerve that transfers visual information to the vision centers of the brain
3	Pericardium (PC)	Oculomotorius	The nerve that innervates four of the six extra-ocular muscles that control movement of the eye
4	Heart (HT)	Trochlearius	The nerve that innervates the superior oblique muscle, which enables looking down and up and rotation in the plane of the face

Cranial nerve number	Chinese medicine organ and channel association to the cranial nerve	Latin name	Western medicine function
5	Stomach (ST)	Trigeminus	The sensory nerve of the face
6	San Jiao (SJ)	Abduceus	The nerve that innervates the muscle that abducts the eye
7	Small Intestine (SI)	Facialis	The nerve that innervates the muscles of the face and salivary glands and transfers sensory information on taste from the anterior two-thirds of the tongue
8	Spleen/Pancreas (PI)	Vestibulocohlearis	The nerve that transfers information about hearing and balance from the ear to the brain
9	Lung (LU)	Glossopharyngeus	A sensory and motor nerve that innervates various structures in the head and neck. It is important in swallowing because it elevates the larynx during swallowing
10	Liver (LIV)	Vagus	The main nerve of the parasympathetic nervous system, and its functions are both motor and sensory
11	Gallbladder (GB)	Accessorius	A motor nerve that innervates the sternocleidomastoid and trapezius muscles
12	Large Intestine (LI)	Hypoglossus	A motor nerve that innervates almost all muscles of the tongue

Bibliography

. . . . . .

Dharmananda, S. and Vickers, E. (2000) *Synopsis of Scalp Acupuncture*. Portland, OR: Institute for Traditional Medicine.

Feely, R.A. (2011) *Yamamoto New Scalp Acupuncture: Principles and Practice* (2nd edn). New York: Georg Thieme Verlag.

Hao, J.J. and Hao, L.L. (2012) "Review of clinical applications of scalp acupuncture for paralysis: An excerpt from Chinese scalp acupuncture." *Global Advances in Health and Medicine 1*, 1, 102–121.

Moore, K.L., Agur, A.M.R. and Dalley, A.F. (2013) *Clinically Oriented Anatomy* (7th edn). Philadelphia, PA: Wolters Kluwer Health/Lippincott Williams & Wilkins.

Wang, S., Liu, K., Wang, Y., He, X. et al. (2017) "A proposed neurologic pathway for scalp acupuncture: Trigeminal nerve–meninges–cerebrospinal fluid–contacting neurons–brain." *Medical Acupuncture 29*, 5, 322–326.

Yamamoto, T. and Yamamoto, H. (1999) *YNSA, Yamamoto New Scalp Acupuncture*. Chiyoda, Japan: Medical Tribune.

Yamamoto, T., Yamamoto, H. and Yamamoto, M.M. (2010) *Yamamoto New Scalp Acupuncture* (2nd edn). Japan: Self-published.

Zeise-Suess, D. (2008) *New YNSA ZS Point for Disturbances of Female Hormonal Systems*. Remchingen, Germany. Available at https://doi.org/10.1089/acu.2007.0610

About the Authors

• • • • • •

David Bomzon, Lic.Ac. is a classical Chinese medicine practitioner and lecturer, and a former student of Dr Toshikatsu Yamamoto, the founder of this technique. He specializes in neurorehabilitation acupuncture and is one of the leading acupuncture therapists in the rehabilitation field in Israel. David has been working for over 10 years in the rehabilitation department of Bnei-Zion medical center, Haifa, Israel. He has led an integrative medicine approach in the rehabilitation department, using scalp acupuncture as one of the rehabilitation tools for the patients. In his work, David combines western medical knowledge with a Chinese medicine approach. He founded the Pnima Center—an Integrative Chinese Medicine Center—in Haifa, Israel in 2007. David is considered an authority on YNSA in Israel and a world-renowned lecturer on this topic.

Avi Amir, Lic.Ac. is a therapist who specializes in Chinese medicine and medical massage therapy, and in particular the treatment of orthopedic problems and pain. He also practices YNSA, which he studied under the guidance of Dr Toshikatsu Yamamoto. Avi is one of the co-founders of the International School of Scalp Acupuncture, and is an active managing partner of the community clinic at the Pnima Center. At Pnima, Avi treats over 150 patients a week using Chinese medicine and medical massage.

Index

• • • • • •

Conditions Index

• • • • • •